Urology
at a Glance

This title is also available as an e-book.
For more details, please see
www.wiley.com/buy/9781118923641
or scan this QR code:

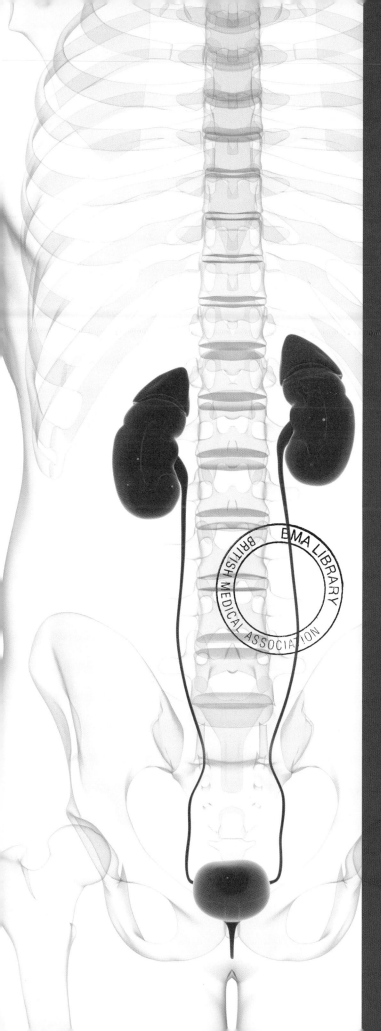

Urology
at a Glance

Edited by

Hashim Hashim

MBBS, MRCS(Eng), MD, FEBU, FRCS(Urol)
Consultant Urological Surgeon in Female,
Functional and Reconstructive Urology
and Director of the Urodynamic Unit, Bristol
Urological Institute, Southmead Hospital,
Bristol, UK
Honorary Senior Lecturer, University of Bristol,
UK

Prokar Dasgupta

MSc(Urol), MD, DLS, FRCS, FRCS(Urol), FEBU
Professor of Robotic Surgery and Urological
Innovation
Guy's Hospital, King's College London, UK

WILEY Blackwell

This edition first published 2017 © 2017 by John Wiley & Sons, Ltd

Registered office:	John Wiley & Sons, Ltd, The Atrium, Southern Gate, Chichester, West Sussex, PO19 8SQ, UK
Editorial offices:	9600 Garsington Road, Oxford, OX4 2DQ, UK
	The Atrium, Southern Gate, Chichester, West Sussex, PO19 8SQ, UK
	111 River Street, Hoboken, NJ 07030-5774, USA

For details of our global editorial offices, for customer services and for information about how to apply for permission to reuse the copyright material in this book please see our website at www.wiley.com/wiley-blackwell

Library of Congress Cataloging-in-Publication Data

Names: Hashim, Hashim, editor. | Dasgupta, Prokar, editor.

Title: Urology at a glance / edited by Hashim Hashim, Prokar Dasgupta.

Other titles: Urology at a glance (Hashim) | At a glance series (Oxford, England)

Description: Chichester, West Susex, UK ; Hoboken, NJ : John Wiley & Sons Inc., 2017. | Series: At a glance series | Includes bibliographical references and index.

Identifiers: LCCN 2016030552| ISBN 9781118923641 (pbk.) | ISBN 9781118923658 (epub)

Subjects: | MESH: Urologic Diseases | Genital Diseases, Male | Diagnostic Techniques, Urological

Classification: LCC RC871 | NLM WJ 140 | DDC 616.6—dc23 LC record available at https://lccn.loc.gov/2016030552

A catalogue record for this book is available from the British Library.

Wiley also publishes its books in a variety of electronic formats. Some content that appears in print may not be available in electronic books.

Cover image: © SEBASTIAN KAULITZKI/GettyImages

Set in Minion Pro 9.5/11.5 by Aptara
Printed and bound in Singapore by Markono Print Media Pte Ltd

1 2017

Contents

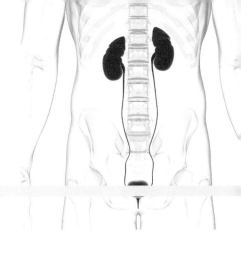

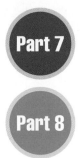

Contributors

Hashim U. Ahmed, Chapter 16
MRC Clinician Scientist and Reader in Urology
Division of Surgery and Interventional Sciences
University College London
London, UK

Waseem Akhter, Chapters 13 and 14
Specialty Registrar in Urology
North West London Trainee
Frimley Health NHS Foundation Trust
Frimley, UK

Salah Al Buheissi, Chapter 5
Consultant Urologist
North Bristol NHS Trust
Bristol, UK

Mo Belal, Chapter 11
Consultant Urological Surgeon
University Hospital Birmingham
Queen Elizabeth Hospital
Birmingham, UK

Michelle Christodoulidou, Chapter 12
Research Fellow in Urology
University College London Hospitals
London, UK

James F. Donaldson, Chapter 15
Speciality Registrar in Urological Surgery
Western General Hospital;
Tutor, MCh in Urology
University of Edinburgh and Royal College of Surgeons
    of Edinburgh
Edinburgh, UK

Hazel Ecclestone, Chapter 18
Urology Registrar
Charing Cross Hospital
London, UK

David S.J. Ellis, Chapter 9
Clinical Fellow in Urology
Imperial College Healthcare NHS Trust
London, UK

Michael S. Floyd (Jr), Chapter 7
Specialist Registrar in Urology
Whiston Hospital
St Helens and Knowsley Teaching Hospitals NHS Trust
Liverpool, UK

Rizwan Hamid, Chapter 18
Consultant Urological Surgeon
University College London Hospitals;
London Spinal Cord Injury Centre, Stanmore, UK

Hashim Hashim, Chapters 1–3
Consultant Urological Surgeon in Female, Functional and
    Reconstructive Urology;
Director of the Urodynamic Unit
Bristol Urological Institute
Southmead Hospital;
Honorary Senior Lecturer
University of Bristol
Bristol, UK

Talal Jabbar, Chapters 4 and 5
Fellow in Female, Functional and Reconstructive
    Urology
Bristol Urological Institute
Bristol, UK

Rozh Jalil, Chapters 13 and 14
Specialty Registrar in Urology
North West London Trainee
Frimley Health NHS Foundation Trust
Frimley, UK

Rahim Kaba, Chapter 8
Specialty Registrar in Urology (STR5)
Stepping Hill Hospital
University College London Hospitals;
London Spinal Injuries Unit, Stanmore, UK

Jas Kalsi, Chapters 12–14
Consultant Urological Surgeon and Andrologist
Imperial College Healthcare
Frimley Health Foundation Trust
Frimley, UK

Abi Kanthabalan, Chapter 16
Clinical Research Fellow
University College London Hospitals NHS Foundation Trust
London, UK

Sachin Malde, Chapter 10
Consultant Urological Surgeon
Guy's and St Thomas' NHS Foundation Trust
London, UK

Asif Muneer, Chapter 12
Consultant Urological Surgeon and Andrologist;
Honorary Senior Lecturer
University College London
London, UK

David Muthuveloe, Chapter 11
Urology Registrar
University Hospital Birmingham
Birmingham, UK

Arie Parnham, Chapter 19
Locum Consultant Urologist
Manchester Royal Infirmary
Manchester, UK;
Honorary Senior Associate Lecturer
Edge Hill University
Ormskirk, UK

Ian Pearce, Chapter 19
Consultant Urological Surgeon
Central Manchester University Hospitals NHS Trust
Manchester, UK

Tina G. Rashid, Chapter 9
Consultant Urological Surgeon
Imperial College Healthcare NHS Trust
London, UK

Mutie Raslan, Chapter 15
Speciality Registrar in Urology
Aberdeen Royal Infirmary
Aberdeen, UK

Justine Royle, Chapter 15
Consultant Urological Surgeon and Associate
    Postgraduate Dean
Aberdeen Royal Infirmary
Aberdeen, UK

Arun Sahai, Chapter 10
Consultant Urological Surgeon and Honorary Senior
    Lecturer
Department of Urology, Guy's Hospital;
MRC Centre for Transplantation, King's College London
London, UK

Matthew Shaw, Chapter 6
Consultant Urological Surgeon
Freeman Hospital
Newcastle upon Tyne, UK

Iqball S. Shergill, Chapter 7
Consultant Urological Surgeon
Wrexham Maelor Hospital, Wrexham, UK;
Honorary Senior Lecturer
Manchester Medical School, University of Manchester,
    Manchester, UK;
Honorary Senior Lecturer
Division of Biological Sciences, University of Chester,
    Chester, UK;
Honorary Clinical Teacher
Cardiff University School of Medicine, Cardiff, UK;
Clinical Director
North Wales and North West Urological Research Centre
    (NW2URC)
University of Chester, Chester, UK

Andrew Sinclair, Chapter 8
Consultant Urologist
Stepping Hill Hospital
Stockport NHS Foundation Trust
Stockport, UK

Rajan Veeratterapillay, Chapter 6
Specialist Registrar in Urology
Freeman Hospital
Newcastle upon Tyne, UK

Christian I. Villeda Sandoval, Chapter 5
Consultant Urologist and Robotic Surgery Coordinator
Hospital General Naval y de Alta Especialidad
(General and Specialties Naval Hospital)
Mexico City, Mexico

Dan Wood, Chapter 17
Consultant in Adolescent and Reconstructive Urology
University College London Hospitals
London, UK

Mussab S. Yassin, Chapters 1–3
Specialist Registrar in Urology
Urology Department
Churchill Hospital, Oxford University Hospitals NHS Trust
Oxford, UK

Preface

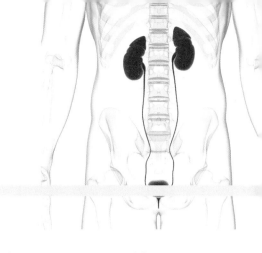

Urology is an exciting specialty incorporating medicine, surgery, paediatrics and the very latest in science and technology. It also continues to evolve rapidly, more perhaps than any other surgical field. We often hear from colleagues, both senior and junior, that it is difficult to keep up with this fast moving pace.

In parallel, the formal teaching of urology itself is facing gentle extinction from many university curricula, particularly in the UK. Many of our medical students are lucky to spend a week on a urology firm, with only the truly interested and the die-hard opting for a urological topic during a Special Study Module or an intercalated BSc. Nevertheless after graduation, most of our students will look after urological patients and therefore need the fundamentals of the specialty on their fingertips.

It is with this mind that we have put together *Urology at a Glance* for your reading pleasure. The majority of authors are UK-based. There is, however, an international flavour as a number are prominent for their important contributions to the growing body of modern literature in high quality journals. The text is deliberately arranged in eight parts to focus the readers minds on their topics of interest.

The book is meant to be an easy reference for medics at all levels of experience. We hope that our readers will find it useful especially when they do not have the time to go through the many encyclopaedic volumes that are out there. Or perhaps when they cannot be entirely certain that Dr Google is giving them the correct information that they need!

We hope you enjoy reading it and welcome your feedback.

Hashim Hashim, Bristol
Prokar Dasgupta, London

About the companion website

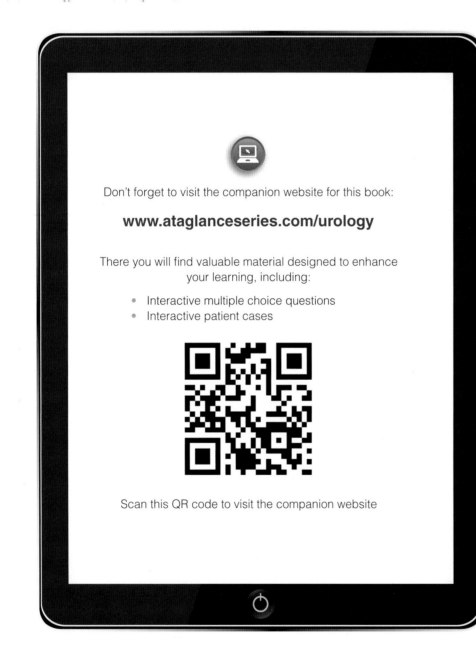

Don't forget to visit the companion website for this book:

www.ataglanceseries.com/urology

There you will find valuable material designed to enhance your learning, including:

- Interactive multiple choice questions
- Interactive patient cases

Scan this QR code to visit the companion website

Urological history, examination and investigations

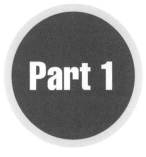

Part 1

Chapters

Taking a urological history

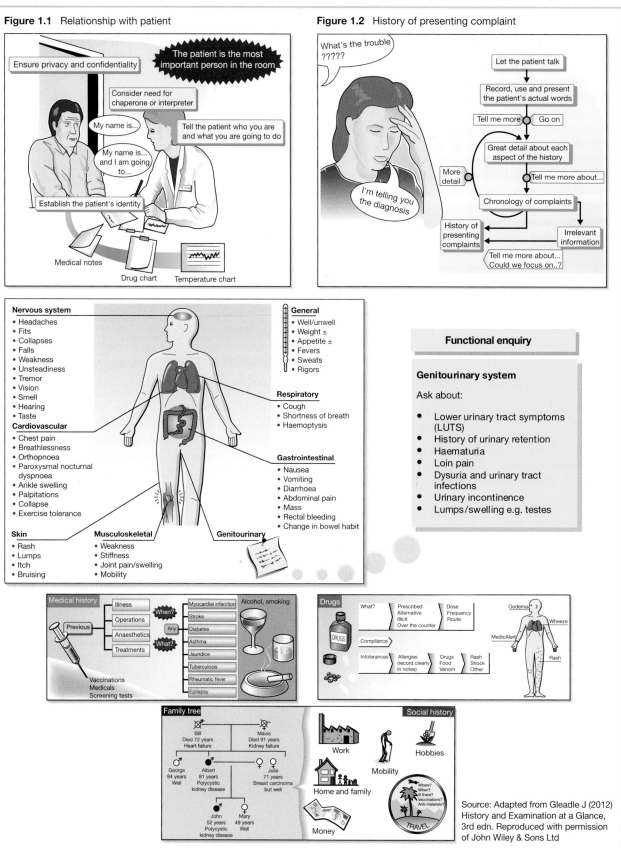

Figure 1.1 Relationship with patient

Ensure privacy and confidentiality

The patient is the most important person in the room

Consider need for chaperone or interpreter

My name is...

Tell the patient who you are and what you are going to do

My name is... and I am going to...

Establish the patient's identity

Medical notes

Drug chart   Temperature chart

Figure 1.2 History of presenting complaint

What's the trouble ?????

I'm telling you the diagnosis

Let the patient talk

Record, use and present the patient's actual words

Tell me more   Go on

Great detail about each aspect of the history

More detail   Tell me more about...

Chronology of complaints

History of presenting complaints

Irrelevant information

Tell me more about... Could we focus on..?

Nervous system
- Headaches
- Fits
- Collapses
- Falls
- Weakness
- Unsteadiness
- Tremor
- Vision
- Smell
- Hearing
- Taste

Cardiovascular
- Chest pain
- Breathlessness
- Orthopnoea
- Paroxysmal nocturnal dyspnoea
- Ankle swelling
- Palpitations
- Collapse
- Exercise tolerance

Skin
- Rash
- Lumps
- Itch
- Bruising

Musculoskeletal
- Weakness
- Stiffness
- Joint pain/swelling
- Mobility

Genitourinary

General
- Well/unwell
- Weight ±
- Appetite ±
- Fevers
- Sweats
- Rigors

Respiratory
- Cough
- Shortness of breath
- Haemoptysis

Gastrointestinal
- Nausea
- Vomiting
- Diarrhoea
- Abdominal pain
- Mass
- Rectal bleeding
- Change in bowel habit

Functional enquiry

Genitourinary system

Ask about:
- Lower urinary tract symptoms (LUTS)
- History of urinary retention
- Haematuria
- Loin pain
- Dysuria and urinary tract infections
- Urinary incontinence
- Lumps/swelling e.g. testes

Medical history
Previous — Illness, Operations, Anaesthetics, Treatments
When? Any What?
Myocardial infarction, Stroke, Diabetes, Asthma, Jaundice, Tuberculosis, Rheumatic fever, Epilepsy
Vaccinations Medicals Screening tests

Alcohol, smoking

Drugs
What? Prescribed Alternative Illicit Over the counter — Dose Frequency Route
Compliance
Intolerances — Allergies (record clearly in notes) — Drugs Food Venom — Rash Shock Other
Oedema Wheeze MedicAlert Rash

Family tree
Bill Died 72 years Heart failure
Mavis Died 91 years Kidney failure
George 84 years Well
Albert 81 years Polycystic kidney disease
Julie 71 years Breast carcinoma but well
John 52 years Polycystic kidney disease
Mary 49 years Well

Social history
Work   Hobbies   Mobility   Home and family   Money   TRAVEL Where? When? Ill there? Vaccinations? Anti-malarials?

Source: Adapted from Gleadle J (2012) History and Examination at a Glance, 3rd edn. Reproduced with permission of John Wiley & Sons Ltd

Urology at a Glance, First Edition. Edited by Hashim Hashim and Prokar Dasgupta. © 2017 John Wiley & Sons, Ltd. Published 2017 by John Wiley & Sons, Ltd.
Companion website: www.ataglanceseries.com/urology

Figure 1.3 History summary

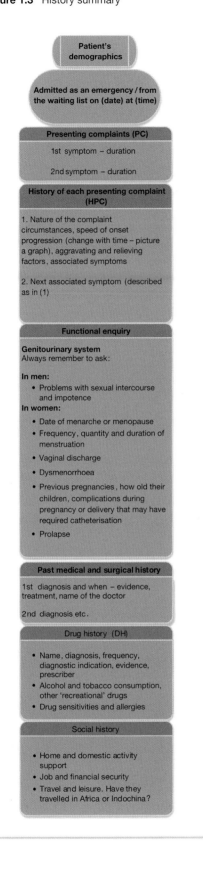

Patient's demographics

Admitted as an emergency / from the waiting list on (date) at (time)

Presenting complaints (PC)

1st symptom – duration

2nd symptom – duration

History of each presenting complaint (HPC)

1. Nature of the complaint circumstances, speed of onset progression (change with time – picture a graph), aggravating and relieving factors, associated symptoms

2. Next associated symptom (described as in (1))

Functional enquiry

Genitourinary system
Always remember to ask:

In men:
• Problems with sexual intercourse and impotence

In women:
• Date of menarche or menopause
• Frequency, quantity and duration of menstruation
• Vaginal discharge
• Dysmenorrhoea
• Previous pregnancies, how old their children, complications during pregnancy or delivery that may have required catheterisation
• Prolapse

Past medical and surgical history

1st diagnosis and when – evidence, treatment, name of the doctor

2nd diagnosis etc.

Drug history (DH)

• Name, diagnosis, frequency, diagnostic indication, evidence, prescriber
• Alcohol and tobacco consumption, other 'recreational' drugs
• Drug sensitivities and allergies

Social history

• Home and domestic activity support
• Job and financial security
• Travel and leisure. Have they travelled in Africa or Indochina?

Relationship with the patient

✓ **Introduction**
Establish the patient identity unequivocally (ask for their full name, date of birth, etc.)

✓ **Privacy**
Ensure that there is privacy (make sure curtains are properly closed; see if the examination room is free)

✓ **Language**
Establish whether they are fluent in the language you intend to use and, if not, arrange for an interpreter to be present

✓ **Relatives, friends, and chaperones**
Establish who else is with them, their relationship with the patient and whether the patient wishes for them to be present during the consultation

✓ **Handwashing**
Hands should be washed before each patient contact with alcoholic rub or medicated soap

History of presenting complaint

This is the most important part of the history. It usually provides the most important information in arriving at the differential diagnosis with vital insight into the complaints that the patient gives the greatest importance to

✓ **Let the patient talk**
The presenting complaint should be obtained by allowing the patient to talk, usually without interruption. Record the history using the patient's own words

✓ **More specific questioning**
Open questions should be addressed to reveal more detail about particular aspects of the history. For example 'Tell me more about the loin pain?'

✓ **Focus on the main problems**
Keep in mind the main problems and direct the history accordingly. It may be necessary to interject and divert the discussion with questions like 'could you tell me more about your loin pain?'

Functional enquiry

✓ An enquiry about the patient sexual activity status and/or sexual gender preferences may be relevant if there are genital or perineal symptoms

✓ An obstetric history is important in a female patient with voiding symptoms

✓ If a patient complaints of LUTS, pneumaturia (passing air with urine which is indicative of colovesical fistula i.e. communication between the bowel and the urinary bladder), haematuria or abdominal pain/lump, then a general enquiry should be made about bowel habit, appetite and weight loss

Drug history

✓ A history of smoking is important in bladder and kidney cancer

✓ Alcohol and caffeine intake might be relevant when considering storage bladder symptoms e.g. frequency or nocturia

✓ Certain drugs can cause chronic cystitis and haematuria e.g. Cyclophosphamide

Social history

✓ Occupation: Ask retired people about their previous occupation especially if they have exposure to rubber, chemicals or plastics. For example, someone complaining of haematuria working for 20 years in a tyre company probably has bladder cancer

✓ Support: Establish whether the patient lives with a responsible and caring adult who could help look after the patient after any operation that might be required

Tip
A drawing can save many words so a sketch noting where the pain starts from and radiates to can be useful, together with a word to specify the type of pain (e.g. sharp, colicky or dull).

2 Male genital examination

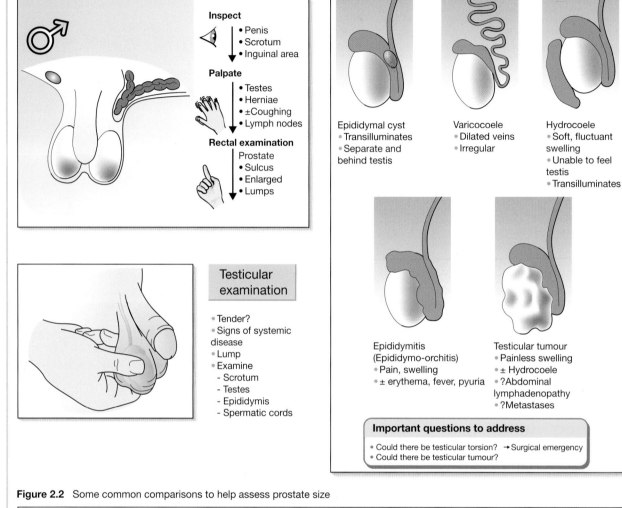

Figure 2.1 Male genital examination
Source: Gleadle J (2012) History and Examination at a Glance, 3rd edn. Reproduced with permission of John Wiley & Sons Ltd.

Inspect
• Penis
• Scrotum
• Inguinal area

Palpate
• Testes
• Herniae
• ±Coughing
• Lymph nodes

Rectal examination
Prostate
• Sulcus
• Enlarged
• Lumps

Testicular examination
• Tender?
• Signs of systemic disease
• Lump
• Examine
 - Scrotum
 - Testes
 - Epididymis
 - Spermatic cords

Epididymal cyst
• Transilluminates
• Separate and behind testis

Varicocoele
• Dilated veins
• Irregular

Hydrocoele
• Soft, fluctuant swelling
• Unable to feel testis
• Transilluminates

Epididymitis (Epididymo-orchitis)
• Pain, swelling
• ± erythema, fever, pyuria

Testicular tumour
• Painless swelling
• ± Hydrocoele
• ?Abdominal lymphadenopathy
• ?Metastases

Important questions to address
• Could there be testicular torsion? → Surgical emergency
• Could there be testicular tumour?

Figure 2.2 Some common comparisons to help assess prostate size

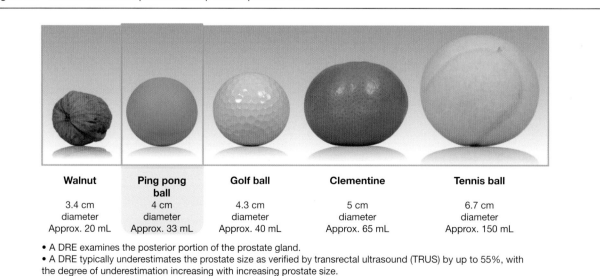

Walnut	Ping pong ball	Golf ball	Clementine	Tennis ball
3.4 cm diameter Approx. 20 mL	4 cm diameter Approx. 33 mL	4.3 cm diameter Approx. 40 mL	5 cm diameter Approx. 65 mL	6.7 cm diameter Approx. 150 mL

• A DRE examines the posterior portion of the prostate gland.
• A DRE typically underestimates the prostate size as verified by transrectal ultrasound (TRUS) by up to 55%, with the degree of underestimation increasing with increasing prostate size.

The penis

Inspection

Note particularly size, shape, presence or absence of a foreskin, colour of the skin, the position and calibre of the urethral meatus, any discharge, abnormal curvature and other superficial abnormality such as erythema or ulceration, particularly at the glans (Figure 2.1).

Palpation

Note any abnormalities of the underlying tissues (e.g. firm areas). This can indicate the plaques of Peyronie's disease. Retract the foreskin to expose the glans penis and urethral meatus. The foreskin should pull back with a smooth and painless retraction. Look especially for any secretion or discharge and collect a specimen if possible. Replace the foreskin to its normal position at the end of the examination.

Key points
- Explain to the patient that you would like to examine the penis and testes and reassure them that the procedure will be quick and gentle.
- You should have a chaperone present.
- Ensure that the examination room is warm and that you are unlikely to be disturbed. With the patient on a bed or couch, raised to a comfortable height, ask them to pull their clothing down. You should be able to see the genitalia and lower part of the patient's abdomen at the very least.

The scrotum and contents

Inspection

This can be carried out with the patient lying down or standing up. Examine the scrotal skin. The left testis usually hangs lower than the right. Remember to lift the scrotum, inspecting the inferior and posterior aspects. Look especially for oedema, sebaceous cysts, ulcers, scabies and scars (Figure 2.1).

Palpation

The scrotal contents should be gently supported with your left hand and palpated with the fingers and thumb of your right hand. It may help to ask the patient to hold their penis to one side. Examine the normal testis first if the patient is complaining of an abnormality in one of them.
- Check that the scrotum contains *two* testes. Absence of one or both testes can be because of previous surgery, failure of the testis to descend or a retractile testis. If there appears to be a single testis, carefully examine the inguinal canal for evidence of a discrete swelling that could be an undescended testis.
- Make careful note of any discrete lumps or swellings in the body of the testis. Any swelling in the body of the testis must be considered to be suggestive of a malignancy.
- Compare the left and right testes, noting the size and consistency. The testes are normally equal in size, smooth, with a firm, rubbery consistency. If there is a significant discrepancy, ask the patient if he has ever noticed this.
- Feel for the epididymis which lies at the posterolateral aspect of each testis.

Scrotal swellings

If a lump is palpable:
- Decide if the lump is confined to the scrotum. Are you able to feel above it? Does it have a cough impulse? Is it fluctuant?

(You will be unable to get above swellings that descend from the inguinal canal.)
- Define the lump and any other mass.
- Transillumination is often important here. Darken the room and shine a small torch through the posterior part of the swelling. A solid mass remains dark while a cystic mass or fluid will transilluminate. If it transilluminates, it would suggest there is a hydrocele.
- Feel for any varicoceles (feels like worms in a bag): the patient should be examined in the lying and standing positions for this to see if it disappears. Varicoceles on the left side warrant a renal scan as well as a scrotal scan.

The local lymphatics

This is best performed with the patient lying comfortably on a bed or couch.
- Lymph from the skin of the penis and scrotum drains to the inguinal lymph nodes.
- Lymph from the covering of the testes and spermatic cord drains initially to the internal, then common, iliac nodes.
- Lymph from the body of the testes drains to the para-aortic lymph nodes. These are impalpable.

The perineum and rectum

Key points in digital rectal examination (DRE)
- Usually performed in the left lateral position – with the patient lying on their left side, and with the hips and knees flexed to 90° or more (if you are right handed).
- Examine the anal region for fistulae and fissures.
- Apply plenty of lubricating gel to the gloved finger.
- Palpate the surface of the prostate. Note its consistency (normal or firm), its surface (smooth or irregular) and estimate its size.

Normal bi-lobed prostate has a groove (the median sulcus) between the two lobes. In the patient with prostate cancer, this groove can be obscured.

The prostate will be very tender if it is involved by an acute, inflammatory condition such as acute, infective prostatitis or a prostatic abscess.

Practical tips
- A normal prostate is the size of a walnut, a moderately enlarged prostate that of a tangerine and a large prostate the size of an apple or orange (Figure 2.2).
- DRE should be avoided in the profoundly neutropenic patient (risk of septicaemia) and in patients with an anal fissure where DRE would be very painful.
- The integrity of the sacral nerves that innervate the bladder and the sacral spinal cord can be established by eliciting the bulbocavernosus reflex (BCR) during a DRE. The sensory side of the reflex is elicited by squeezing the glans of the penis. The motor side of the reflex is tested by feeling for contraction of the anus during this sensory stimulus.

Further reading

Gleadle J. *History and Clinical Examination at a Glance*, 3rd edn. Oxford: Wiley-Blackwell; 2012.

Resnick MI, Novick AC. *Urology Secrets*, 3rd edn. Philadelphia, PA: Hanley & Belfus; 2002.

Thomas J, Monaghan T. *Oxford Handbook of Clinical Examination and Practical Skills (Oxford Medical Handbooks)*. Oxford: Oxford University Press; 2007.

3 Female genital examination

Figure 3.1 Digital bimanual vaginal examination:
(a) bimanual palpate areas 1, 2, 3 in order; (b) digital bimanual palpation of the pelvis.

(a)

Uterus between abdominal and vaginal examining fingers

(b)

Symphysis pubis
Empty bladder

Tender, red, fluctuant mass
• Occur in the labia minora / labia majora fold at 5- or 7-o'clock positions
• Major symptoms are fever and acute unilateral vulvar pain

(c)

Figure 3.1 (c) Bimanual examination of the adnexa
• The two fingers of the vaginal hand are moved into the deep right vaginal fornix
• The abdominal hand is placed just medial to the anterior superior iliac spine
• The two hands are brought as close together as possible and the adnexa is palpated with a single motion

Figure 3.2 Cusco's speculum examination

(a) Speculum enters vagina closed with opening mechanism pointing to patient's right

(b) Speculum is inserted deeply, rotated 90° then opened

(c) Cervix comes into view once speculum is opened

Figure 3.3 Sim's speculum examination of the vaginal walls

Figure 3.4 Types of pelvic organ prolapse

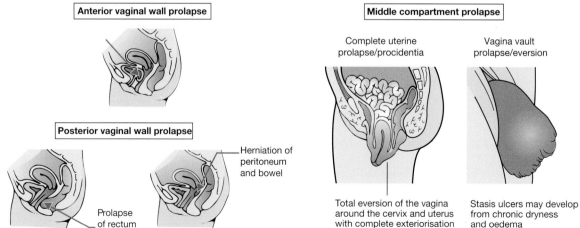

Anterior vaginal wall prolapse

Posterior vaginal wall prolapse

Prolapse of rectum

Herniation of peritoneum and bowel

Middle compartment prolapse

Complete uterine prolapse/procidentia

Vagina vault prolapse/eversion

Total eversion of the vagina around the cervix and uterus with complete exteriorisation

Stasis ulcers may develop from chronic dryness and oedema

Source: Figures 3.1-3.3 Impey L, Child T. (2012) Obstetrics and Gynaecology, 4th edn. Reproduced with permission of John Wiley & Sons Ltd. Figure 3.4 Norwitz E & Schorge J (2013) Obstetrics and Gynaecology, 4th edn. Reproduced with permission of John Wiley & Sons Ltd.

Urology at a Glance, First Edition. Edited by Hashim Hashim and Prokar Dasgupta. © 2017 John Wiley & Sons, Ltd. Published 2017 by John Wiley & Sons, Ltd.
Companion website: www.ataglanceseries.com/urology

Examination of the external genitalia

Inspection

Uncover the mons to expose the external genitalia making note of the pattern of hair distribution. Apply a lubricating gel to the examining finger. Separate the labia from above with the forefinger and thumb of your left hand. Inspect the clitoris, urethral meatus for stenosis (rare) or urethral caruncles, and vaginal opening. Look especially for any discharge, redness, ulceration, atrophy or old scars. Ask the patient to cough or strain down and look at the vaginal walls for any prolapse and assess for any leakage of urine. Also look at the mobility of the urethra. Ask the patient to squeeze as if she is trying to stop passing urine to look for pelvic floor lift.

Palpation

Palpate the length of labia majora between the index finger and thumb. The tissue should feel pliant and fleshy. Palpate for Bartholin's gland with the index finger of the right hand just inside the introitus and the thumb on the outer aspect of the labium majora (Figure 3.1).

Bartholin's glands are only palpable if the duct becomes obstructed resulting in a painless cystic mass or an acute Bartholin's abscess. The latter is seen as a hot, red, tender swelling in the posterolateral labia majora.

Speculum examination

There are different types of vaginal specula but the most common is the Cusco's speculum which allows inspection of the cervix and vaginal walls (Figure 3.2) and the Sims' speculum which

Key points

- Explain to the patient that you would like to examine them and reassure them that the procedure will be quick and gentle.
- Ensure the abdomen is covered. Ensure good lighting and remember to wear disposable gloves.
- You should have a chaperone present.
- Ensure that the room is warm and well lit, preferably with a moveable light source and that you will not be disturbed.
- The patient should be allowed to undress in privacy and, ideally have a comfortably full bladder.
- Ask the patient to lie on her back on an examination couch with both knees bent up and let her knees fall apart either with her heels together in the middle or separated.
- Warm the speculum under running water and lubricate it with a water-based lubricant.
- Using the left hand, open the lips of the labia minora to obtain a good view of the introitus.
- Hold the speculum in the right hand with the main body of the speculum in the palm and the closed blades projecting between index and middle fingers.
- Gently insert the speculum into the vagina held with your wrist turned such that the blades are in line with the opening between the labia.
- The speculum should be angled downwards and backwards due to the angle of the vagina.
- Maintain a posterior angulation and rotate the speculum through 90° to position the handles anteriorly.
- When it cannot be advanced further, maintain a downward pressure and press on the thumb piece to hinge the blades open exposing the cervix and vaginal walls.
- Once the optimum position is achieved, tighten the thumbscrew.
- Removing the speculum should be conducted with as much care as insertion. You should still be examining the vaginal walls as the speculum is withdrawn.
- Undo the thumbscrew and withdraw the speculum. The blades should be held open until their ends are visible distal to the cervix to avoid causing pain.
- Rotate the open blades in an anticlockwise direction to ensure that the anterior and posterior walls of the vagina can be inspected.
- Near the introitus allow the blades to close, taking care not to pinch the labia or hairs.

Table 3.1 Oxford scale for grading pelvic floor muscle strength (Laycock & Jerwood 2001). Description: index finger 4–6 cm inside vagina at 4 and 8 o'clock positions with moderate pressure

Grade	Muscle contraction strength (denoted by P for power in acronym)	
0	Nil	Nil
1	Flicker	Flicker
2	Increase in tension, no discernible lift	Weak
3	Lift of muscle belly and elevation of post vaginal wall / indrawing of perineum	Good
4	Good contraction / elevation of posterior vaginal wall against resistance	Moderate
5	Strong resistance to elevation of post vaginal wall / finger drawn into vagina	Strong

allows better inspection of the vaginal walls and is used in particular if prolapse is suspected (Figure 3.3). Examination with the Sims' speculum is undertaken with the patient in the left lateral position with legs curled up, while for an examination with Cusco's speculum the patient lies as for the digital examination.

Findings

Inspect the cervix, which is usually pink, smooth and regular. Look for cervical erosions which appear as strawberry-red areas spreading circumferentially around the os and represent extension of the endocervical epithelium on to the surface of the cervix. Identify any ulceration or growths which suggest cancer. Cervicitis can cause a mucopurulent discharge associated with a red, inflamed cervix which bleeds on contact. Take swabs for culture if discharge is seen.

Bimanual examination (per vaginum or PV exam)

Digital examination helps identify the pelvic organs.
- Ideally, the bladder should be emptied, if not already done so by this stage. The patient should be positioned as described before.
- Expose the introitus by separating the labia with the thumb and forefinger of the gloved left hand.
- Gently introduce the lubricated index and middle fingers of the right hand into the vagina.
- Insert your fingers with the palm facing laterally and then rotate 90° so that the palm faces upwards.
- The thumb should be abducted and the ring and little finger flexed into the palm.
- To assess the pelvic floor strength, the women is asked to squeeze her pelvic floor and the strength of contraction is graded according to the Oxford grading system (Table 3.1).

Rectal examination

A rectal examination is sometimes required, particularly if there is posterior wall prolapse (Figure 3.4) or malignant cervical disease.

Practical tip

Atrophic vaginitis is diagnosed clinically in postmenopausal women with labial dryness, loss of skin turgidity and smooth, shiny vaginal epithelium. Treatment options include topical oestrogens.

Further reading

Hogen Esch F, Whelan M, Morin M, Thompson J. State of the art pelvic floor muscle assessment – which tool should we use? ICS Workshop. www.ics.org/workshops/handoutfiles/000197.pdf (accessed 14 July 2016).

Impey L, Child T. *Obstetrics and Gynecology*, 4th edn. Oxford: Wiley-Blackwell; 2012.

Norwitz ER, Schorge JO. *Obstetrics and Gynecology at a Glance*, 4th edn. Oxford: Wiley-Blackwell; 2013.

4 Urological investigations

Figure 4.1 IVU full-length image taken after 15 min showing filling defects (tumour) in bladder over left side causing mild left hydronephrosis

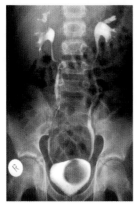

Figure 4.2 CT urogram showing the excretory phase within the pelvicalyceal system of both kidneys. Filling defect in the right renal pelvis (arrow) could represent a urothelial tumour of the renal pelvis

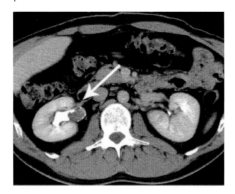

Figure 4.3 TRUS biopsy of prostate: (a) the anatomical relations of the prostate and the path for the passage of biopsy needle through the ultrasound probe into the prostate; (b) horizontal view of the prostate

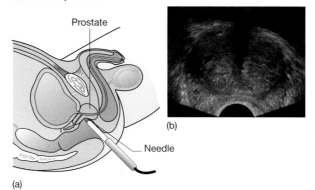

(b)

Prostate

Needle

(a)

Figure 4.4 Urine flow meter and commode with the printing machine to show electronic traces of the flow

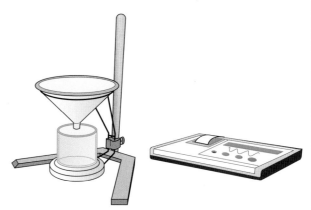

Figure 4.5 Urodynamic trace showing incontinence caused by detrusor overactivity

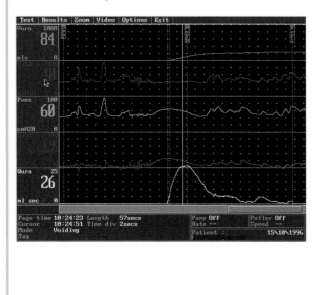

Figure 4.6 Technetium-99m MAG3. The images were acquired with the patient's back facing the camera. The left kidney is on the reader's left. Upper left panel shows 20 sequential 2-s dynamic flow images showing the initial bolus of activity travelling down the abdominal aorta into both kidneys. Upper right panel shows the regions of interest used to correct for background and used to generate the renogram curves. The curves peak by 5 min and show rapid washout of the tracer from the kidneys. The time to peak height for both kidneys is 2.7 min. The 20 min/maximum and 20 min/2–3 min activity ratios also are displayed

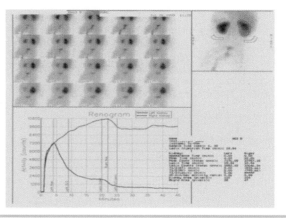

Urology at a Glance, First Edition. Edited by Hashim Hashim and Prokar Dasgupta. © 2017 John Wiley & Sons, Ltd. Published 2017 by John Wiley & Sons, Ltd.
Companion website: www.ataglanceseries.com/urology

Radiology departments make a crucial contribution to the diagnosis of urological conditions and to their treatment, in the form of interventional radiology. Imaging of the urinary tract provides information on anatomy, function, and frequently both, as well as showing pathological lesions. In most instances a combination of imaging modalities will be required to provide the information needed to plan the most appropriate form of management. The choice of imaging modality will be based on the presenting clinical problems, patient factors, availability of techniques and whether treatment is available. Some of the imaging tests come at the cost of radiation exposure; hence it is important to keep the radiation burden to the patient as low as possible, especially in high-risk groups such as children, pregnant women, young patients and patients with renal impairment.

The most commonly used radiological tests in urology are a plain radiograph of kidney–ureter–bladder (KUB), ultrasound (US), computed tomography (CT) and magnetic resonance imaging (MRI). Intravenous urography (IVU) is now performed only infrequently and on a very selective basis.

However, there are other investigations to assess the function of the lower or upper urinary tract. Flow rate tests and urodynamic studies are used for assessment of function of the lower urinary tract, while dimercaptosuccinic acid (DMSA) and mercaptoacetyltriglycine (MAG3) renograms can be used to assess the function of the upper tract.

Intravenous urogram/pyelogram

Although the IVU has largely been replaced by CT urogram, it retains a limited role in providing information in certain specific areas such as:

- Delineating the level of an acute obstruction (e.g. from calculi) with limited images following non-contrast CT KUB to minimise the radiation to the patient and avoid a further CT urogram
- Further assessment of distal ureters with limited images, if the CT scan is inconclusive, to avoid taking the patient to the operating theatre to perform a cystoscopy and retrograde ureteropylogram under general anaesthetic.

IVU involves ionising radiation: 3–4 films of IVU is equivalent to 100 times the dose from a chest X-ray, which has a minimal radiation dose (2.5 mSv).

The patient should be asked about any allergies or previous adverse reactions to contrast materials and iodine. IVU should not routinely be performed in patients with renal impairment as the contrast will not be excreted sufficiently to provide good images and it can cause further deterioration in renal function.

The number and sequence of films taken varies between radiology departments, the indication for the test and patient factors. A typical sequence of images would be:

- Control film (KUB) X-ray
- Full-length image taken 5 minutes after contrast injection
- An image of the kidney at 15 mintues (Figure 4.1)
- Further full-length image
- Post micturition image.

CT urogram

CT has a high ionising radiation dose; however, it is widely available, is a relatively quick test, does not need a radiologist and provides more accurate information than US or IVU with diagnosis of non-urological problems. Non-contrast CT KUB is now considered the first-line investigation for any patient with suspected renal colic.

CT urogram (radiation dose 10–15 mSv) carries much higher radiation exposure to patients than non-contrast CT KUB (radiation dose 3.5–4.5 mSv), although it provides much more significant information about the whole urinary tract including any renal, pelvicalyceal system, ureteric or even bladder lesions. Every effort should be made to make sure that it is correctly indicated and to keep the radiation dose to a minimum.

Intravenous access is required for the injection of contrast material. Again, all precautions before using contrast should be applied, such as any history of allergy to iodine, renal function, pregnancy status in women, diabetic patients on metformin (the main concern would be potential precipitation of lactic acidosis with accumulation of metformin, which is exclusively excreted via the kidneys) and severe asthma.

The common sequences of a CT urogram are pre-contrast, vascular phase and excretory phase (Figure 4.2) to show the pelvicalyceal systems, ureters and bladder. The availability of multi-detector helical and multi-slice CT allows the acquisition of much faster and multiple slices per cube rotation with 3D reconstruction which has increased the accuracy of diagnosis of urological conditions and reduces the timing for each CT scan to accommodate more patients per session.

Transrectal ultrasound scan and biopsy of prostate

TRUS is an ultrasound technique used to scan the prostate, seminal vesicles, surrounding tissues and any congenital lesions within the prostate such as Müllerian duct cysts. The ultrasound transducer (probe) sends sound waves through the wall of the rectum into the prostate gland, which is located directly in front of the rectum (Figure 4.3). Rectal probes are available in side and end-fire models with transmission frequencies of 7.5 MHz. It remains a first-line investigation for raised prostate-specific antigen (PSA) and other prostatic abnormalities in most urology departments at the present time.

A TRUS is usually performed as an outpatient procedure under local anaesthesia (LA) if a biopsy is being taken from the prostate. If the patient is unable to tolerate the procedure under LA, then it can be performed under general anaesthesia in theatre. The test usually takes 15–30 minutes. There are a few preparations for the patient before performing the procedure:

- Informed consent – explaining the risk and problems which can be very serious such as infection, prostatitis, septicaemia, rectal bleeding, haematuria, haematospermia, chronic pelvic pain syndrome or chronic prostatitis and urinary retention
- Antibiotic prophylaxis according to local microbiology policy
- Rectal swab, enema or laxative – not routine practice by all departments, but depends on local protocols
- Digital rectal examination
- Peri-prostatic LA (e.g. 10 mL 1% lignocaine)
- Complete evaluation of prostate in both transverse and sagittal sections
- Measurement of prostate volume with or without PSA dynamic test such as PSA density
- Biopsy of prostate using a spring-driven 18-gauge needle core biopsy device or gun (usual number of cores is 12, with 6 from each side).

As can be seen, it is an invasive procedure and carries risk, so all patients should be counselled appropriately with clear indications for the procedure:

- Measurement of prostate size, and to exclude congenital abnormalities of the prostate – if this is the only indication, no biopsy is taken and no LA is required
- Diagnose prostate cancer
- Raised PSA, abnormal DRE or other abnormalities detected on other imaging modalities such as CT or MRI

- Part of active surveillance protocol for men with low-risk prostate cancer who wish to avoid radical treatment such as radical prostatectomy or radical radiotherapy
- To guide the placement of implants during brachytherapy treatment or to guide cryotherapy or high-intensity focused ultrasound (HIFU) treatment of prostate.

Flow rate test or uroflowmetry

This is an important non-invasive measurement to assess the voiding pattern in patients with LUTS, normally represented graphically and reported in terms of variables such as maximum flow rate (Qmax), voided volume and trace pattern. There are three physical principles for different types of flow meter machines: weight transducer, rotating disc and capacitance flow meters (Figure 4.4). The flow rate is dependent on several factors to interpret it accurately: age and gender of the patient, voided volume, the pressure generated in the bladder and the resistance caused by the prostate or urethra. A simple flow rate measurement cannot be used to accurately distinguish the difference between a weak bladder (detrusor underactivity during voiding) or bladder outflow obstruction (for instance caused by prostate enlargement, stricture or failure of the sphincter to relax during voiding) without pressure measurement of the bladder while the patient is voiding.

Clear instructions or an information leaflet should be sent out to patients in advance of the flow test. They should be informed of the need to attend the urology department for 2–3 hours, having a comfortably full bladder after drinking 500 mL to 1 L of fluid. Two or three flow rate measurements will be performed on the same day, and male patients have to avoid compressing the penis or squeezing the pelvic floor (squeeze artefact), avoid moving the area around the funnel of flow meter (wag/cruising artefact) and avoid moving the machine (knock artefact).

There are various types of flow pattern that indicate problems in the function of the lower urinary tract. The normal patterns are bell-shaped, but a compressive pattern could indicate bladder outflow obstruction caused by prostate enlargement or a prolapse in women, a plateau pattern could be consistent with a stricture and intermittent interrupted flow could indicate straining caused by detrusor underactivity.

Urodynamics

In contrast to flow rate tests, urodynamics (UDS) describes both the physiology of the storage–filling phase and the voiding phase of the urinary cycle, and also the measurement of the strength of the urethral sphincter using urethral pressure profile measurement. Therefore, UDS assesses changes in the pressure in the bladder and urethra. Typically, the aim of UDS is to reproduce the patient's symptoms in a controlled fashion, and to perform an evaluation of storage–filling and voiding phases of micturition (Figure 4.5).

There are different types of UDS based on clinical indications and the patient's history. The commonly performed UDS tests are standard without imaging or fluoroscopy and video-urodynamics which include performing retrograde cystogram during filling to assess bladder morphology or the presence of ureteric reflux, then to perform micturating cystogram during the voiding phase with pressure measurement during all phases. Another type is the ambulatory UDS which can be carried out if the previous two tests fail to indicate the cause for the patient's symptoms.

UDS is a diagnostic test, analogous to an electrocardiogram (ECG) in the heart. It can help to predict the effects of lower urinary tract dysfunction on the upper tract, outcome and sequelae of treatment, confirm therapeutic effects and understand the reasons for previous failed therapeutic interventions.

Although it is perceived to be somewhat invasive by patients, serious complications related to UDS testing are extremely rare, with an infection rate of about 2–3%.

The International Continence Society (ICS) has described criteria for various UDS findings including bladder outflow obstruction (BOO), detrusor overactivity or underactivity and impaired compliance. Therefore, these are UDS terms, although they have been used in clinical practice without UDS findings which can cause confusion so adherence to correct terminology is very important.

Dimercaptosuccinic acid (DMSA) renogram and mercaptoacetyltriglycine (MAG3) renogram

DMSA is a static renography test that involves technetium-99m. DMSA binds to the convoluted tubules of the kidney, with only 10% of the injected dose being excreted by the kidney. It provides static images of functioning renal tissue and generates a measure of relative rather than absolute renal function. DMSA provides information about the presence and progression of renal scarring and is the modality of choice for identifying atrophic, poorly functioning or ectopic/horseshoe kidneys and other congenital renal anomalies. It is one of the common imaging tests used in children with recurrent urinary tract infections (UTIs).

The MAG3 renogram is a dynamic renography test which involves technetium-99m. It relies on tubular excretion and thus is a diagnostic investigation for obstruction of kidney drainage. Dynamic renograms allow simultaneous assessment of renal function and drainage (Figure 4.6).

For both tests, split renal function of each kidney, or even each moiety in case of duplex anomaly, can be acquired. Both tests use a gamma camera and non-ionising radiation so have a low risk of radiation. Images are obtained by drawing regions of interest around each kidney and one or more suitable background regions. Patients should be well hydrated as they sit in front of the gamma camera and should avoid contact with pregnant women or young children afterwards. Patients will remain radioactive for 4–6 hours, but are not a significant hazard (Table 4.1).

Table 4.1 Comparison of DMSA and MAG3 tests

DMSA	MAG3
Static test	Dynamic test
Bound to technetium-99m isotope	Bound to technetium-99m isotope
Small percentage excreted by the kidney and the rest is deposited in the tubular cells of the kidney	Most excreted by the kidney
Used to investigate presence of renal scarring or presence of renal tissues especially in congenital abnormalities + split renal function	Used to investigate obstruction + split renal function
Uses gamma camera	Uses gamma camera
Takes 2–4 hours	Takes 30–40 minutes

Further reading

Challacombe B, Bott S. *Diagnostic Techniques in Urology*. London: Springer; 2014.

Rao NP, Srinangam SJ, Preminger GM. *Urological Tests in Clinical Practice*. London: Springer; 2007.

Reynard J, Brewster S, Biers S. *Oxford Handbook of Urology*, 3rd edn. Oxford: Oxford University Press; 2013.

5 Abdominal pain

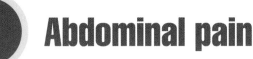

Box 5.1 PQRST mnemonic for pain assessment

P3	Positional, palliating (alleviating) and provoking factors
Q	Quality
R3	Region, radiation, referral
S	Severity
T3	Temporality (onset, progression, previous episodes)

Box 5.2 Neurological pathways for abdominal pain

- Stimulation of autonomic nerves invested in the visceral peritoneum surrounding internal organs
- Pain is porly characterised and difficult to localise
- Upper abdominal pain: foregut – stomach, duodenum, liver and pancreas
- Periumbilical pain: midgut – small bowel, proximal colon and appendix
- Lower abdominal pain: hindgut – distal colon and genitourinary tract
- Irritation of the parietal peritoneum, sensations are conducted by peripheral nerves
- Pain is better localised
- Stimulation through peripheral afferent nerves from some internal organs when they enter the spinal cord through nerve roots that also carry nociceptive fibres from other locations
- Sensation felt at a distance from its source

Figure 5.1 Primary localisation of pain according to its origin

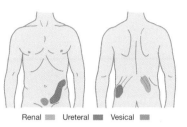

Renal ▩ Ureteral ▩ Vesical ▩

Figure 5.2 Bimanual examination of the kidney

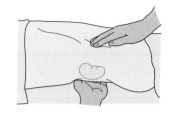

Figure 5.3 Bimanual examination of the bladder in male and female patients

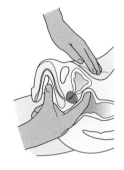
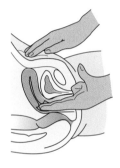

Box 5.3 Types of abdominal pain and their anatomical locations

Renal pain	Usually located in the ipsilateral costovertebral angle beneath the 12th rib; it radiates across the flank anteriorly and can be referred to the testis or labium
Ureteric pain	Can be located in the ipsilateral lower quadrants of the abdomen when originated in its superior segment and can produce bladder storage symptoms and suprapubic discomfort when coming from the inferior portion; it can also refer to the scrotum or labium
Bladder pain	Usually suprapubic, although it can refer to the distal urethra and the urethral meatus
Penile pain	Usually referred from the bladder or urethra; primary causes are paraphimosis, priapism or Peyronie's disease when related to erections
Scrotal pain	Can be referred from the upper urinary tract, while primary origin usually arises within the scrotum and its contents and, interestingly, can be referred to ipsilateral lower abdominal quadrants

Figure 5.4 Plain KUB showing bilateral renal stones

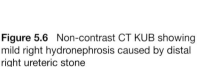

Figure 5.5 Ultrasound of the kidney showing dilatation of renal pelvis and calyces

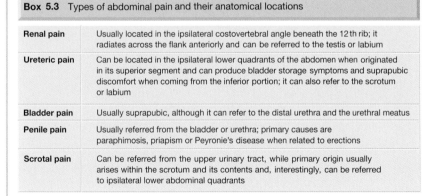

Box 5.4 Common urological causes of abdominal pain

1. Renal/ureteric colic with or without obstruction
2. Pyelonephritis
3. Urine retention
4. Bladder stones
5. Urinary tract infections
6. Painful bladder syndrome/interstitial cystitis
7. Chronic pelvic pain syndrome
8. Acute or chronic prostitis
9. Testicular torsion
10. Renal abscess
11. Renal infarction or renal vein thrombosis
12. Retroperitoneal bleeding or haematoma

Figure 5.6 Non-contrast CT KUB showing mild right hydronephrosis caused by distal right ureteric stone

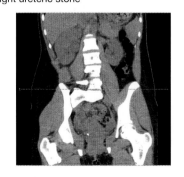

Urology at a Glance, First Edition. Edited by Hashim Hashim and Prokar Dasgupta. © 2017 John Wiley & Sons, Ltd. Published 2017 by John Wiley & Sons, Ltd.
Companion website: www.ataglanceseries.com/urology

Abdominal pain is the most common reason for a visit to the emergency department, accounting for approximately 7–10% of total visits. It remains one of the most challenging presentations for any doctor. As urologists, we tend to narrow our differential diagnosis to our familiar spectrum of diseases. However, it is important to keep in mind all the possible differential diagnoses and to perform a full assessment of the patient without any prejudgement biases.

As ever, history and physical examination are the main pillars of the differential diagnosis construct. Medical, surgical and social histories provide important additional information. Always consider the most likely and obvious explanations first, but never forget to keep an open mind for less common diseases.

When faced with a patient in pain, history-taking should be quick, effective and concise (Box 5.1). Making a correct diagnosis is a dynamic process which evolves as we go through the history, physical examination and diagnostic tests. Age and gender are the first filters to discriminate amongst possible differential diagnoses. Then, having in mind the patient's background, a detailed assessment of the pain is the next step. Severity and temporality allow further narrowing of the options.

The origin of abdominal pain can be suggested by its characteristics, which differ according to the neurological pathway that translates and carries the stimuli (Box 5.2). In urology, abdominal pain usually originates from the retroperitoneal compartment. Hence, having localised anterior or peritonitic abdominal pain usually makes a urological condition unlikely. Another useful hint is that a patient with retroperitoneal pain is restless and moves around, while one with intraperitoneal pathology usually lies motionless.

Pain arising from the genitourinary tract is usually severe when produced by obstruction or inflammation. Urinary calculi can cause excruciating pain when obstructing the ureter, but can be asymptomatic in the bladder or renal pelvis despite being of considerable size. Inflammation in pyelonephritis, prostatitis and epididymitis creates capsular distention, and is usually severely painful. Inflammation of mucosal layers usually produces moderate discomfort as with cystitis or urethritis. Pain localisation, radiation and referral suggest its anatomical origin (Box 5.3; Figure 5.1).

Physical examination

Physical examination is the first diagnostic test for patients with abdominal pain. A patient with abdominal pain will always appreciate gentle movements and objective explanations as well as precise and steady manoeuvres (Box 5.4).

The kidneys

The kidneys are difficult to palpate as they are hidden behind the protective ribcage. However, the most common method is with the patient positioned in the supine or lateral position during deep inspiration. With one hand the kidney is lifted or pushed from the posterior wall of the abdomen below the costovertebral angle and the other hand pushes in the anterior abdominal wall below the costal margin (Figure 5.2). The kidney or any lesion fixed to it move with respiration unlike fixed retroperitoneal masses. Gentle percussion over the costovertebral angle can confirm pain arising from a distended or inflamed renal capsule when poorly localised pain is referred by the patient.

The bladder

The bladder can only be palpated when holding more than 300 mL in an adult. A distended bladder holding 500 mL or more is easily palpable in a non-obese patient. Percussion can help to identify the dullness of a distended bladder surrounded by resonant bowel contents. A bimanual examination can help to identify possible tumours in the bladder, but it is preferably performed under sedation or anaesthesia. The bladder is palpated between the abdomen and vagina in the female or the abdomen and rectum in the male (Figure 5.3).

The scrotum

The scrotum and its contents can be examined using the fingertips of both hands. The testes are normally round, firm and smooth and 6 × 4 cm in length and width. The epididymis lies posteriorly and is palpated as a soft ridge. The testes should be noted for size and consistency. Any hard area should be considered malignant until proven otherwise; however, epididymal masses are almost certainly benign.

Transillumination of a large scrotal mass can support the diagnosis of a hydrocele if it transilluminates easily; a solid tumour is not translucent. Transillumination is usually performed with a torch pen which is shone through a small solid tube placed perpendicularly on the scrotal skin in a darkened room. Alternatively, the torch pen can be placed directly on the scrotal skin on one side and transillumination observed from the other side.

In a patient with acute scrotal pain, the absence of the cremasteric reflex, which is elicited by stroking your fingers on the patient's inner thigh after warning them and observing if the testis pulls upwards, can suggest testicular torsion; scrotal pain that subsides with scrotal elevation suggests epididymitis, while persistent pain suggests testicular torsion.

The spermatic cord and groin

The spermatic cord and groin are examined in the standing position with the aid of a Valsalva manoeuvre. A varicocele is a tortuous, dilated vein palpated around the cord. Inguinal hernias can be palpated as a bulge invading or descending into the inguinal canal. The patient's 'normal' side is examined first (i.e. the one that is not causing the problem).

Prostate digital rectal examination

Prostate DRE can be useful to confirm the clinical diagnosis of acute prostatitis when an exquisite pain is elicited and a fluctuant mass is palpated, which can indicate a prostatic abscess. A gentle examination is recommended in this setting. Prostate size can be estimated with little accuracy but more accurate measurement of prostate size can be ascertained during TRUS or MRI scan.

The consistency of the prostate is more important and whether it has a smooth surface suggestive of benign enlargement or a hard craggy feeling indicative of malignancy. Palpation of hard nodule or discrepancy in the feeling of any lobes of the prostate can also indicate malignancy. Clinical staging of prostate cancer is based on DRE findings.

Examination of the anterior abdomen

This is essential to rule out differential diagnoses arising from intraperitoneal organs; therefore generalised tenderness and guarding indicate peritonitis and palpation of a central expansile pulsatile mass should raise the alarm for a leaking aortic aneurysm. Localised tenderness with guarding and rebound tenderness over the right iliac fossa could be related to acute appendicitis.

Diagnostic tests

The diagnosis of acute abdominal pain in urology can be supported by specific tests. The aim of these examinations must be to confirm one of the previous working diagnoses suggested during interrogation and physical examination. Nowadays, plain abdominal radiography, ultrasonography and CT imaging are the most favoured tests. IVP is no longer commonly used in modern practice.

X-ray KUB

A plain abdominal X-ray must include kidneys, ureters and bladder (KUB) and the diaphragm down to the inferior border of the symphysis pubis (Figure 5.4). Although it has lost popularity since the advent of the CT scan, KUB is still useful for evaluating urinary stone disease, especially in patients with known radio-opaque stones. It is also valuable to assess the position and location of catheters and stents placed after urological procedures.

Ultrasound

Ultrasonography of the urinary tract can expedite imaging of the kidneys, bladder and scrotum which is accessible at the side of the patient. It is widely available and relatively non-expensive. It provides useful images without ionising radiation and is not dependent on the patient's renal function to provide improved imaging, so it is the imaging modality of choice for special populations such as children, pregnant women and patients with acute kidney injury or chronic kidney disease.

Renal ultrasound in the emergency department is useful to rule out upper urinary tract obstruction in the collecting systems in the form of hydronephrosis (Figure 5.5). It is defined as distention of the renal calyces and pelvis with urine as a result of obstruction of the outflow of urine distal to the renal pelvis. Although its sensitivity to identify the specific cause such as stones, strictures or tumours is limited, confirming obstruction will prompt further investigations and ruling it out with the absence of hydronephrosis will avoid them. Mild hydronephrosis or isolated distention of the renal pelvis without the calyxes can yield a significant number of false positive results, but calyx dilatation is definitely a significant finding.

Ureteric dilatation can occasionally be identified and implies more distal obstruction, but likewise further investigation is usually required. Peri-renal and renal lesions >2 cm such as abscesses and tumours can also be confidently identified with this technique.

Ultrasonography is an operator-dependent assessment and obesity, intestinal gas and physical deformity can be a relative impediment for a substantive evaluation. Ultrasonography can also be used to evaluate the pelvis. A common cause for emergency evaluation in urology is acute urinary retention. Despite being a clinical diagnosis on most occasions, a full bladder can be difficult to evaluate in patients with morbid obesity or body habitus abnormalities. In patients with haematuria, a large blood clot can be confirmed if suspected because of unresolved haematuria or continuous catheter blockage.

Occasionally, abdominal pelvic ultrasound is required to rule out other causes of pain, especially in young female patients with suprapubic pain.

Testicular ultrasound in the emergency setting is not generally used for acute testicular pain as most clinicians support prompt surgical decision-making, particularly when an acute scrotum is suspected.

CT scan

Multi-detector helical CT is the current imaging modality of choice for acute abdominal pain. A non-contrast CT scan has higher than 90% sensibility and specificity for urinary tract stones, hydronephrosis and can also provide further information about renal and retroperitoneal tumours, fluid collections and abscesses. It is a useful tool to ratify a suspected diagnosis, but also provides further information in cases when a differential diagnosis must be additionally investigated. The main disadvantages of this technique is the exposure to ionising radiation and, although widespread nowadays, it is more expensive than and not as accessible as other simpler techniques. The patient must be stable to be transported and undergo the CT scan although portable CT scanners are now available.

A CT scan provides useful anatomical information (Figure 5.6) unlike any of the previously mentioned modalities. A simple rule of thumb for the authors of this chapter is to choose ultrasound scan when the aim is to rule out potentially life-threatening complications in the emergency department. However, when the aim is to confirm a diagnosis and a potential intervention is likely, a CT scan will provide more information if it is accessible and no contraindications exist.

Further reading

Clavijo-Eisele J (ed.) *Handbook of On Call Urology*. Grimsby: Urology Solutions; 2015.

Japp AG, Robertson C (eds). *Macleod's Clinical Diagnosis*. Churchill Livingstone; 2013.

McLatchie G, Borley N (eds). *Oxford Handbook of Clinical Surgery*, 4th edn. Oxford: Oxford University Press; 2013.

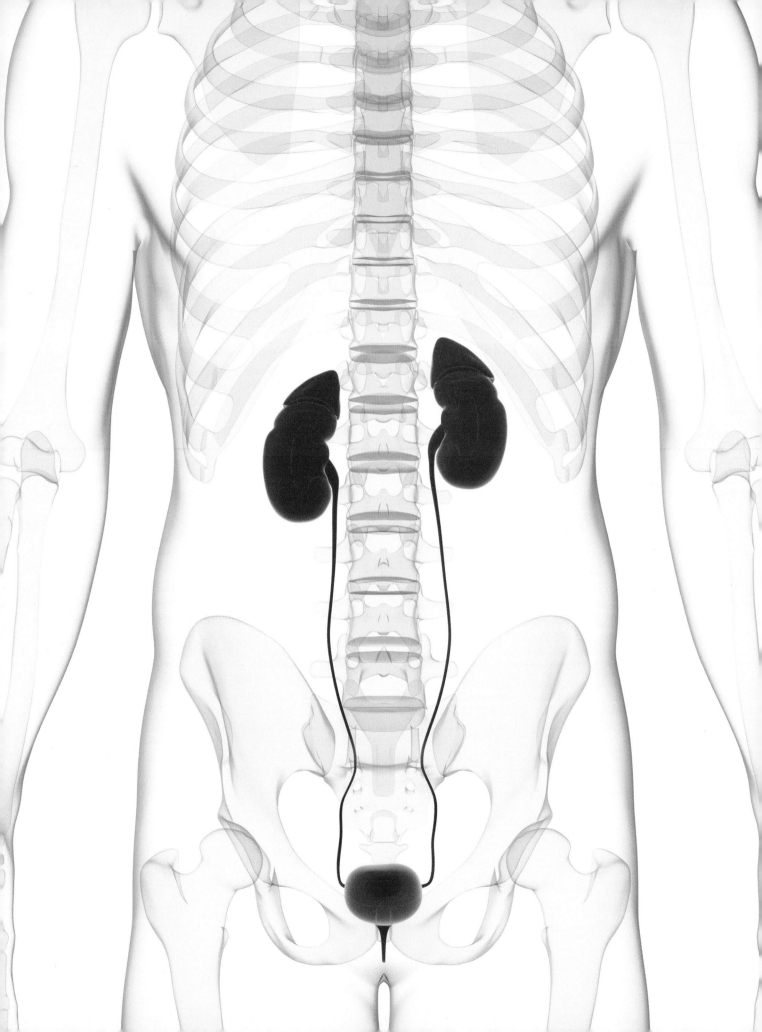

Kidney and ureter

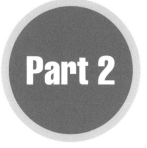

Part 2

6 Urolithiasis

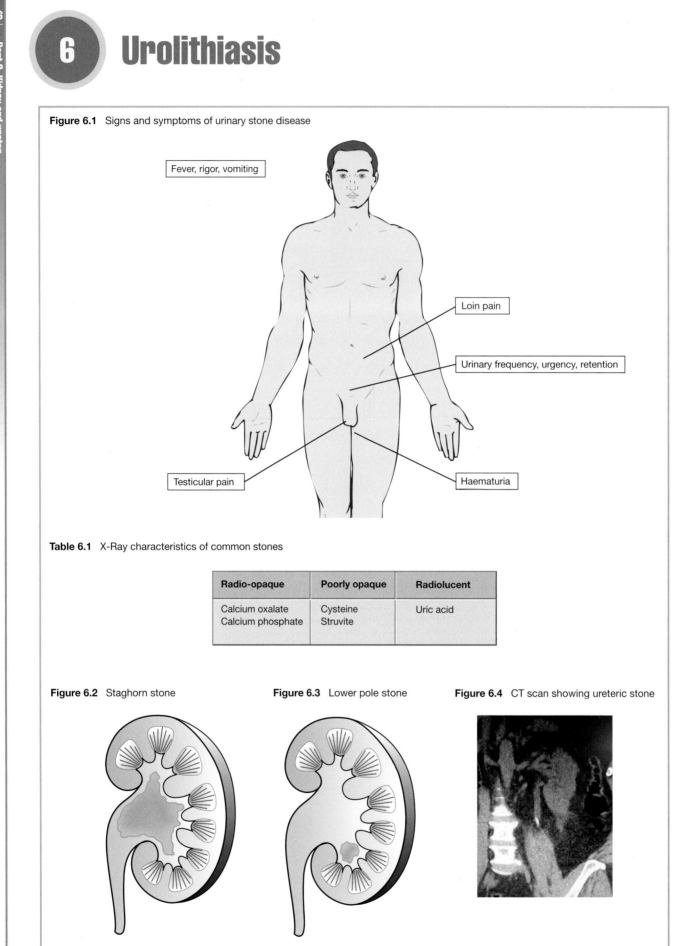

Figure 6.1 Signs and symptoms of urinary stone disease

Fever, rigor, vomiting

Loin pain

Urinary frequency, urgency, retention

Testicular pain

Haematuria

Table 6.1 X-Ray characteristics of common stones

Radio-opaque	Poorly opaque	Radiolucent
Calcium oxalate Calcium phosphate	Cysteine Struvite	Uric acid

Figure 6.2 Staghorn stone

Figure 6.3 Lower pole stone

Figure 6.4 CT scan showing ureteric stone

Urology at a Glance, First Edition. Edited by Hashim Hashim and Prokar Dasgupta. © 2017 John Wiley & Sons, Ltd. Published 2017 by John Wiley & Sons, Ltd.
Companion website: www.ataglanceseries.com/urology

Urinary tract stone disease is an increasing problem, influenced by patient and environmental factors. The prevalence of stones is up to 7%, with the peak incidence occurring at 20–50 years. Males are three times more likely to be affected than females, with stones occurring more commonly in Caucasian and Asian patients. It is likely that dietary factors, such has increased protein consumption and reduced fluid intake, coupled with sedentary occupations increase the risk of stone disease. Urinary tract stones present in many ways (Figure 6.1).

Types of stones

Stones can be classified according to size, location, composition, aetiology or X-ray characteristics.

Composition

There aremarked sex and regional variations in stone composition, but most stones are calcium-based. Calcium oxalate account for up to 70%, mixed calcium oxalate/phosphate 10% and calcium phosphate 5–10%. Non-calcium stones include uric acid 7–10%, struvite (infection) 6% and cystine 0.5%. Rarer stones can be caused by drugs such as indinavir and triamterene.

X-ray characteristics

Stones can appear as radio-opaque, poorly radio-opaque or radiolucent. Table 6.1 shows the types of stones and their appearance on X-ray imaging.

Aetiology of stone types

With careful assessment it is possible to identify a predisposing factor behind most urinary tract stones.

Calcium oxalate stones

Hypercalciuria occurs in 30–60% of calcium stone oxalate formers. There are three types: absorptive (intestinal hyperabsorption of calcium leads to a high renal filtered load), renal (impaired renal reabsorption of calcium) and resorptive (increased reabsorption of calcium from bone due to several factors including elevated parathyroid hormone (PTH)).

Hypocitraturia is found as an isolated cause of calcium stones in 5%. It acts to prevent formation of crystals of calcium oxalate and calcium phosphate.

Hyperoxaluria is caused by dietary excess, enteric factors (malabsorption of calcium in the gut in situations of bowel resection or inflammatory bowel disease causes excess oxalate absorption from the bowel) and primary hyperoxaluria (due to autosomal recessive abnormality of glyoxalate metabolism causing an excess of oxalate production).

Hyperuricosuria causes a nidus of uric acid crystal facilitating the formation of calcium oxalate crystals.

Calcium phosphate stones

These stones occur in patients with renal tubular acidosis which occurs as a result of the kidney's ability to acidify urine. The high urine pH facilitates the precipitation of calcium and phosphate as stones.

Uric acid stones

Uric acid is a product of purine metabolism. At a urine pH of <5.5 most uric acid exists in its insoluble undissociated form which is the main constituent of a uric acid stone. As the pH of urine increases the soluble monosodium urate crystals form which reduces the risk of urate stone formation, but increases the chance of making calcium oxalate and calcium phosphate stones. Human urine is usually acidic. Gout predisposes to uric acid stone formation, with up to 20% of those with gout forming uric acid stones.

Myeloproliferative disease and the use of cytotoxic drugs increase the risk of uric acid stones because of a high filtered load of uric acid from the release of cellular nucleic acids from the process of cell death.

Struvite stones

These stones are also known as infection stones or triple phosphate stones. They are made up of magnesium ammonium phosphate, often in association with calcium apatite. A high urine pH (>7.2) and the presence of ammonia from the action of a urea-splitting bacteria is required. Urea is broken down by a urease enzyme produced by the bacteria to form ammonia and CO_2 resulting in the alkaline environment required for the precipitation of magnesium ammonium phosphate. Many bacteria possess the urease enzyme, including *Proteus mirabilis, Klebsiella pneumoniae, Pseudomonas* species and *Staphylococcus aureus*. Women have a higher rate of urinary tract infection than men, which in part explains struvite stones being more common in women.

Cystine stones

An autosomal recessive abnormality of a dibasic amino acid transporter in the membrane of cells in the intestine and proximal tubule results in a failure of reabsorption of cystine from the urine. Cystine is insoluble in urine, particularly acidic urine, and readily forms stones.

Presentation of urolithiasis

Urinary tract stone disease can be discovered incidentally by imaging studies performed for other conditions. However, stones can manifest a variety of symptoms (Figure 6.1) including pain and haematuria, both visible and non-visible. In addition, patients with struvite stones can present with infection or fever. Urinary urgency or frequency can result from stone in the lower ureter and occasionally symptoms of renal failure from obstructive uropathy can be manifest.

Assessment – acute

The thorough assessment of a patient with urolithiasis should establish the correct diagnosis, identify the septic patient with a stone and rule out other life-threatening scenarios such as a ruptured abdominal aortic aneurysm or appendicitis.

An effective medical history can establish previous stone disease, factors predisposing to urolithiasis or an alternative diagnosis. A careful physical examination and bedside observations will identify alternative potential disease processes and provide evidence of sepsis. Basic laboratory investigations should include urine dipstick analysis (including pH) with

Figure 6.5 Extracorporeal lithotripsy machine

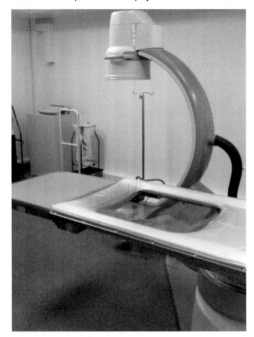

Figure 6.8 Percutaneous nephrolithotomy

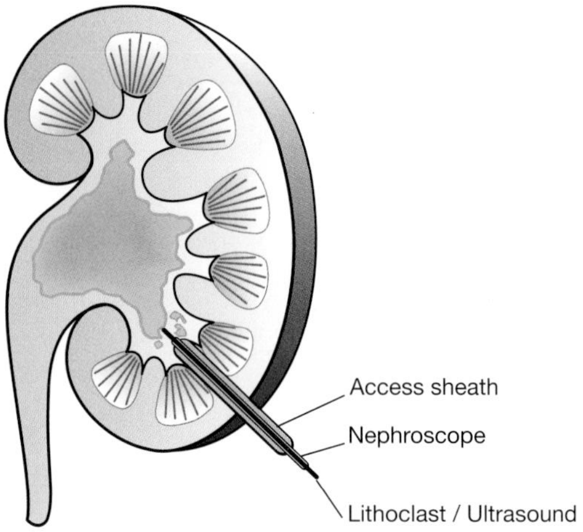

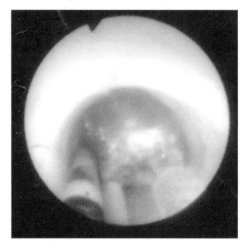

Access sheath

Nephroscope

Lithoclast / Ultrasound

Figure 6.6 Rigid ureteroscopes

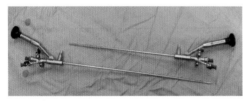

Figure 6.9 Laser fragmentation of ureteric stone

Figure 6.7 Flexible ureteroscope

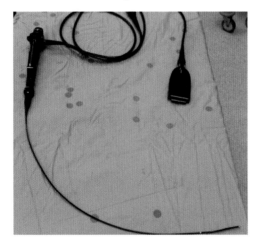

microscopy and culture if sepsis is suspected. Haematuria is noted in 95% of patients with acute stone disease within the first 12 hours of symptoms. In female patients of child-bearing age a pregnancy test should be performed after gaining permission. Biochemical assessment should include sodium, potassium, creatinine, ionised calcium, uric acid and C-reactive protein (CRP). A full blood count (FBC) is required.

Imaging is required to establish the diagnosis of urinary tract stone disease. A non-contrast CT (NCCT) scan of the urinary tract has become the standard imaging modality for acute flank pain. The sensitivity of this study is 96–100% and specificity is 92–100%, and is superior to IVU. An NCCT will show stone location, size and density while also potentially identifying alternative pathology in the absence of stones (Figures 6.2–6.4). Alternative imaging modalities include plain abdominal radiography which is useful in the ongoing monitoring of stone status, but up to one-third of stones are not visible with this technique. Intravenous urography gives useful information on calyceal anatomy, but again will not positively identify radiolucent stones and poses a small risk of contrast allergy. Renal ultrasound is highly sensitive (95%) for renal stones, but is affected by patient body habitus and is much less sensitive for ureteric stones.

Management – acute

Analgesia

If possible the use of non-steroidal anti-inflammatory drugs (NSAIDs) is advocated for analgesia as they offer good analgesic efficacy and patients require less additional analgesia in the short term. In situations where NSAIDs are contraindicated or ineffective then opiates are appropriate. The use of NSAIDs has been shown to reduce the risk of further ureteric colic in the current stone episode, with the same being true of some alpha-receptor blockers such as daily tamsulosin.

Observation of ureteral stones

Provided the patient becomes comfortable and there are no signs of sepsis or renal function compromise then it may be appropriate to observe the stone for spontaneous passage. The characteristics of a stone that make it likely to pass have not entirely been defined. It is the case that smaller stones presenting more distally in the ureter are more likely to pass than larger stone presenting proximally. Overall, it looks like a stone of <5 mm has nearly a 70% chance of spontaneous passage over a 40-day period. Medical expulsive therapy using an alpha-blocker, in a meta-analysis has been show to improve the stone passage rate by relaxing ureteral smooth muscle in stones <10 mm. However, in the recent SUSPEND randomised placebo controlled trial, this has been shown not to be the case and therefore medical expulsive therapy with alpha-blockers or calcium channel blockers is no longer recommended.

Intervention for ureteric stones

Indications to intervene include fever or sepsis, uncontrolled pain or evidence of deteriorating renal function. In addition, failure to pass the stone with time or certain social reasons (airline pilots cannot fly with stones *in situ*) prompt intervention.

Intervention for ureteric stones can be either temporising (decompression of the kidney, but with no attempt to remove the stone) or definitive (stone removal). The management of sepsis with an obstructed kidney requires active patient resuscitation and antibiotic use, but also demands surgical decompression as a matter of urgency. This can be either the placement of a percutaneous nephrostomy catheter under local anaesthesia or positioning of a retrograde ureteric stent which most often is performed under general anaesthesia. There is little evidence to support any one technique as superior over the other. It is important to defer definitive treatment of the stone until the sepsis has fully resolved.

The definitive treatment of a ureteric stone is with either ureteroscopy or extracorporeal shock wave lithotripsy (ESWL; Figures 6.5 and 6.6). The choice between the two techniques depends upon stone factors, patient factors and the availability of both techniques. It is likely that ureteroscopy has a better stone-free rate, but a higher risk of complications than ESWL – this must be discussed with the patient. Ureteroscopy is recommended over ESWL in large (>10 mm) proximal ureteric stones; however, for smaller stones (<10 mm) ESWL would be first choice. In the distal ureter, large stones (>10 mm) are best treated with ureteroscopy (Figure 6.9); smaller stones can be treated by either modality.

Management of renal stones

Symptomatic renal stones usually require treatment unless there are contraindications such as significant co-morbidity. Asymptomatic stones are more difficult and decisions to treat are made on factors such as the likelihood of the stone becoming symptomatic, risk to the patient if the stone were to become symptomatic (solitary kidney) and the chance of treatment being successful. There are many treatment strategies for renal stones.

Observation of renal stones

The natural history of renal stones is poorly defined. There is limited information as to what happens to small asymptomatic stones, with studies showing an intervention rate of 11–49% over 4–5 years. Furthermore, evidence that removing small, asymptomatic stones prevents future symptoms or the need for intervention is weak. It is reasonable to observe small, asymptomatic stones for signs of pain, infection, growth or obstruction. Uric acid stones may be suitable for oral chemolysis. Uric acid is most soluble in an alkaline pH, therefore alkalinisation of the urine with an oral agent such as alkaline citrate or sodium bicarbonate can dissolve the stone. In this situation monitoring of the urine pH and serum electrolyte values is recommended.

Extracorporeal shockwave lithotripsy

ESWL involves the application of focused shockwaves on to a stone to produce fragmentation. It can be performed as an outpatient procedure and in certain situations can produce excellent results. ESWL is contraindicated in pregnancy, uncorrected bleeding diathesis and vascular aneurysm formation in or very close to the path of the shockwaves.

The effectiveness of ESWL depends upon the size and composition of the stone, anatomy of the kidney and the ease with which the stone is seen by the lithotripter. Large (>2 cm), hard stones (calcium oxalate monohydrate and cystine) respond poorly to ESWL, particularly if the drainage of the stone fragments is likely to be poor (dependent calyx of kidney).

It is common to see blood in the urine after this treatment and analgesia is usually required. Repeated treatments can be required and some stones do not fragment effectively. Occasionally, significant renal haemorrhage can occur or stone fragments cause urinary tract obstruction.

Flexible ureterorenoscopy

The development of small diameter, flexible ureteroscopes coupled with the advent of holmium laser technology has allowed the retrograde treatment of renal stones (Figure 6.7). Flexible ureterorenoscopy (FURS) can treat stones where ESWL fails such as hard, lower pole stones. Overall, FURS has a higher stone-free rate than ESWL and has advantages in situations of difficult anatomy and obesity. FURS does require general or regional anaesthesia, can be limited by strictures of the ureter and is less successful with a large stone burden which may necessitate multiple treatment episodes.

Percutaneous nephrolithotomy

Percutaneous nephrolithotomy (PCNL) involves the dilatation of a track between the skin and a renal calyx to allow the passage of operating instruments to fragment and remove stone (Figure 6.8). A variety of energy sources can be used to fragment stones including ballistic, ultrasound or laser lithotripsy.

PCNL has the advantage of effectively treating a large stone burden, but is more invasive than ESWL or FURS. Complications of PCNL are mainly related to infection or bleeding from the puncture site. Bleeding is usually effectively managed by selective renal artery angiography and embolisation. Rarely, abdominal or chest organ injury can occur along the track of the procedure.

Open or laparoscopic renal surgery

Open or laparoscopic surgery for stones in a functioning kidney is rarely performed because of the success of the less invasive techniques described earlier. However, in situations where endoscopic treatment has failed or complex anatomical arrangements prevent endoscopic access then open techniques can be required.

Laparoscopic surgery is used most commonly in non-functioning kidneys where either the stone is symptomatic or is likely to cause complications; in this situation a laparoscopic nephrectomy can be the simplest and most effective option.

Metabolic evaluation

All patients should receive the basic laboratory investigation outlined in Chapter 4. Further metabolic assessment is based upon the patient being at high risk of further stone formation or of a serious outcome from stone recurrence. Factors that lead to high risk include (not exhaustive): multiple stone episodes, stones in childhood, positive family history, gastrointestinal disease, abnormal renal tract anatomy, chronic infection and solitary functioning kidney.

High-risk patients should have an additional biochemical assessment of 24-hour urine collection performed at least 20 days after passage or removal of a stone in the acute setting. This assessment should include calcium, oxalate, citrate, uric acid and cystine. Additional studies are guided by the composition analysis of any removed stones.

General lifestyle advice

There is a significant risk of further stone formation; 50% of men with a calcium oxalate stone will form another within 10 years. This risk can be reduced by certain dietary manipulations.

Patients should be advised to drink enough fluid to produce a urine output of 2–2.5 L/day. They should consume a balanced diet rich in vegetables and limited in both animal proteins and salt. Patients should be advised not to restrict calcium intake below normal. Adequate physical activity is recommended and a normal body mass index (BMI) should be maintained.

Further reading

Donaldson JF, Lardas M, Scrimgeour D, et al. Systematic review and meta-analysis of the clinical effectiveness of shock wave lithotripsy, retrograde intra renal surgery and percutaneous nephrolithotomy for lower pole renal stones. *Eur Urol* 2014; 66(5): 612–616.

Keoghane S, Walmsley B, Hodgson D. The natural history of untreated renal tract calculi. *BJU Int* 2010; 105(12): 1627–1629.

Pickard R, Starr K, Maclennan G, et al. Medical expulsive therapy in adults with ureteric colic: a multicentre, randomised, placebo-controlled trial. *Lancet* 2015; 386: 341–349.

7 Renal failure

Figure 7.1 Classification of renal failure

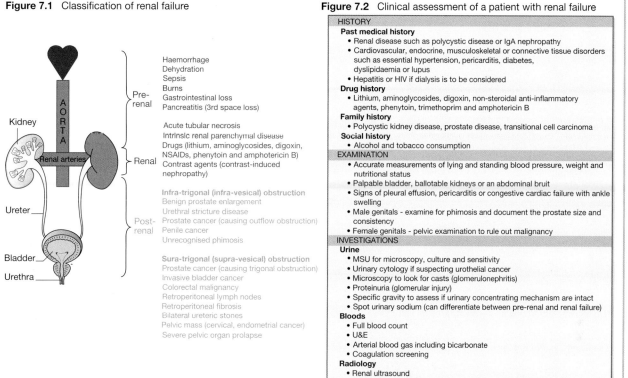

Pre-renal
Haemorrhage
Dehydration
Sepsis
Burns
Gastrointestinal loss
Pancreatitis (3rd space loss)

Renal
Acute tubular necrosis
Intrinsic renal parenchymal disease
Drugs (lithium, aminoglycosides, digoxin, NSAIDs, phenytoin and amphotericin B)
Contrast agents (contrast-induced nephropathy)

Post-renal
Infra-trigonal (infra-vesical) obstruction
Benign prostate enlargement
Urethral stricture disease
Prostate cancer (causing outflow obstruction)
Penile cancer
Unrecognised phimosis

Sura-trigonal (supra-vesical) obstruction
Prostate cancer (causing trigonal obstruction)
Invasive bladder cancer
Colorectal malignancy
Retroperitoneal lymph nodes
Retroperitoneal fibrosis
Bilateral ureteric stones
Pelvic mass (cervical, endometrial cancer)
Severe pelvic organ prolapse

Figure 7.2 Clinical assessment of a patient with renal failure

HISTORY

Past medical history
- Renal disease such as polycystic disease or IgA nephropathy
- Cardiovascular, endocrine, musculoskeletal or connective tissue disorders such as essential hypertension, pericarditis, diabetes, dyslipidaemia or lupus
- Hepatitis or HIV if dialysis is to be considered

Drug history
- Lithium, aminoglycosides, digoxin, non-steroidal anti-inflammatory agents, phenytoin, trimethoprim and amphotericin B

Family history
- Polycystic kidney disease, prostate disease, transitional cell carcinoma

Social history
- Alcohol and tobacco consumption

EXAMINATION
- Accurate measurements of lying and standing blood pressure, weight and nutritional status
- Palpable bladder, ballotable kidneys or an abdominal bruit
- Signs of pleural effusion, pericarditis or congestive cardiac failure with ankle swelling
- Male genitals - examine for phimosis and document the prostate size and consistency
- Female genitals - pelvic examination to rule out malignancy

INVESTIGATIONS

Urine
- MSU for microscopy, culture and sensitivity
- Urinary cytology if suspecting urothelial cancer
- Microscopy to look for casts (glomerulonephritis)
- Proteinuria (glomerular injury)
- Specific gravity to assess if urinary concentrating mechanism are intact
- Spot urinary sodium (can differentiate between pre-renal and renal failure)

Bloods
- Full blood count
- U&E
- Arterial blood gas including bicarbonate
- Coagulation screening

Radiology
- Renal ultrasound
- CT (unenhanced) may be used in certain circumstances
- CT with contrast or IVU are NOT used in contemporaty practice

Figure 7.3 Blood results showing post-renal cause of renal failure

Clinical information: Acute urinary retention

Note that the creatinine level at presentation is extremely elevated at 385 micromol/L

EG	eGFR and electrolytes (AUTHORISED [A])				
NA	Sodium	137		mmol/L	133-146
K	Potassium	3.9		mmol/L	3.5-5.3
CREAT	Creatinine	385		umol/L	H 58–110
EGFR	Estimated GFR	14		ml/min/1.7m2	
	AKI Alert	Acute Kidney Injury Alert. Creatinine increase over baseline value.			
CRP	C-reactive protein (CRP) (AUTHORISED [A])				
CRP	C-reactive protein (CRP)	17		mg/L	H <5
UREA	Urea (AUTHORISED [A])				
Urea	Urea	10.5		mmol/L	H 2.5–7.8

The creatinine: Urea ratio is >10:1 indicating post-renal cause

Date and time collection	CREAT umol/L
13 Nov 2011 08:40	77
28 May 2015 19:01	*385
29 May 2015 00:00	*282
31 May 2015 09:50	*137

Creatinine is significantly higher than the baseline in 2011

The renal function improves after urethral catheterisation, thus confirming a case of post-renal renal failure (obstructive uropathy)

Figure 7.4 Renal ultrasound scan showing bilateral hydronephrosis

There is widespread dilatation of all renal calyces and the renal pelvis bilaterally. Note also that the renal cortex is well maintained – indicating relatively acute onset hydronephrosis, rather than chronic long standing obstruction.

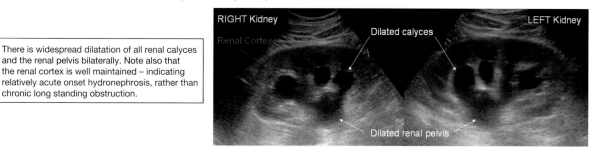

Urology at a Glance, First Edition. Edited by Hashim Hashim and Prokar Dasgupta. © 2017 John Wiley & Sons, Ltd. Published 2017 by John Wiley & Sons, Ltd.
Companion website: www.ataglanceseries.com/urology

Figure 7.5 Anatomical basis for post-renal obstructive uropathy

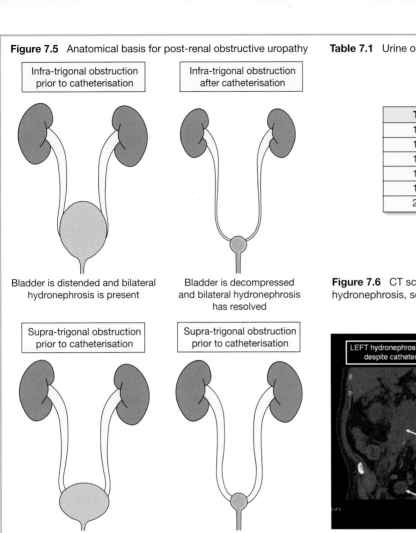

Infra-trigonal obstruction prior to catheterisation

Infra-trigonal obstruction after catheterisation

Bladder is distended and bilateral hydronephrosis is present

Bladder is decompressed and bilateral hydronephrosis has resolved

Supra-trigonal obstruction prior to catheterisation

Supra-trigonal obstruction prior to catheterisation

Normal bladder but bilateral hydronephrosis is present

Bladder is decompressed and bilateral hydronephrosis still remains

Table 7.1 Urine output chart in post obstructive diuresis

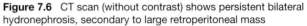

Time	Urine output
15:00	410 mL
16:00	385 mL
17:00	435 mL
18:00	375 mL
19:00	410 mL
20:00	360 mL

Figure 7.6 CT scan (without contrast) shows persistent bilateral hydronephrosis, secondary to large retroperitoneal mass

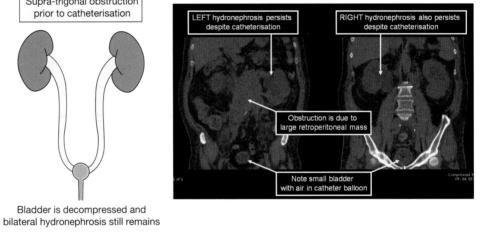

LEFT hydronephrosis persists despite catheterisation

RIGHT hydronephrosis also persists despite catheterisation

Obstruction is due to large retroperitoneal mass

Note small bladder with air in catheter balloon

Classification

Renal failure classification (Figure 7.1) is clinically useful, because pre-renal and renal causes are usually managed medically (nephrologists), and post-renal causes are typically managed by urologists. Post-renal causes result from urinary tract obstruction (obstructive uropathy) or dysfunction. Importantly, it must be understood that several causes can coexist. For example, the urologist who is called to see a patient in retention (post-renal renal failure) will also establish if there are pre-renal causes, like hypovolaemia (as the patient desperately avoids drinking to limit how much urine is produced, so that his bladder does not distend further) and renal causes, including stopping nephrotoxic medications. Interestingly, while the definitive management of post-renal renal failure usually requires urological surgery, most cases can be initially managed by straightforward interventions by junior staff (e.g. simple urethral catheterisation in cases of urinary retention).

Clinical assessment

A thorough and detailed history is mandatory (Figure 7.2). Specific urological questions should focus on abdominal and loin pain, lower urinary tract symptoms (recent deterioration, haematuria or dysuria). Full physical examination is required (Figure 7.2). From the urological perspective, examine for a palpable and percussable bladder. In men, look for phimosis and penile masses, and assess the prostate for size and consistency. In females, a vaginal examination is mandatory to rule out a pelvic mass or malignancy.

Investigations

Urgent U&Es will establish the diagnosis. Typically, as a rule of thumb, a creatinine to urea ratio of >10 : 1 will invariably indicate a post-renal cause (Figure 7.3). Comparison with previous baseline readings can be useful. Raised potassium levels (>5.5 mmol/L) can coexist, and constitute a medical emergency requiring immediate treatment. High serum urea levels and metabolic acidosis on arterial blood gas (ABG) can indicate the need for emergency dialysis. A coagulation screen is required if dialysis or nephrostomy insertion is required urgently. It is not useful – its mandatory.

For the urologist, the presence of hydronephrosis on ultrasound scanning (USS) will strongly indicate a post-renal cause for renal failure (Figure 7.4). Importantly, the presence of a distended bladder will also differentiate the type of obstruction present. There is absolutely no role for contrast CT scan or IVU in the acute setting because of the risk of contrast deteriorating the renal function even further.

Clinical management

Initially, urinary catheterisation is required, and the residual volume needs to be documented. Hourly output measurements should be commenced to assist in determining the type of obstruction, the presence of post-obstructive diuresis, as well as predicting the need for subsequent urological intervention.

Types of post-renal obstruction

Only bilateral urinary obstruction will result in renal failure. In unilateral cases, mechanisms are in place whereby the contralateral (non-obstructed) kidney compensates, resulting in overall normal renal function.

In post-renal renal failure from bilateral urinary obstruction, the anatomical distinction between infra-trigonal (infra-vesical) and supra-trigonal (supra-vesical) will need to be established quickly (Figure 7.5), as this determines correct and effective management. The trigone is the specialised area at the base of the bladder into which the ureters insert. Infra-trigonal obstruction is usually as a result of bladder outlet obstruction, and relief of obstruction from catheterisation will result in resolution of the renal failure (Figure 7.5). However, with supra-trigonal obstruction, catheterisation will not make any difference to the renal failure as the obstructing cause is higher than this level (Figure 7.5).

Post-obstructive diuresis

In cases of post-renal renal failure, relief of urinary obstruction can result in post-obstructive diuresis (POD).

POD is defined as excess urine output at a rate of >200 mL/hour for more than two consecutive hours (Table 7.1). Importantly, in POD there is both a physiological and pathological component to the diuresis. The physiological diuresis occurs as a result of fluid, electrolytes and waste products, accumulated during the preceding period of renal failure, being eliminated 'normally' after relief of obstruction. This diuresis is 'normal' and as such does not necessarily need to be replaced. Critically, pathological diuresis occurs because of tubular dysfunction and inappropriate NaCl/water handling by the kidney, with decreased re-absorption of NaCl by the thick ascending limb of the loop of Henle and decreased re-absorption of urea by the collecting tubule. Crucially, this pathological aspect is abnormal and, as such, the fluid lost does need to be replaced. As the pathological diuresis results in loss of sodium, chloride and water mainly, if POD is diagnosed, the ideal fluid replacement is 0.9% saline. Fluid replacement regimens vary, but a logical value of 50% of the patient's previous hour's urine output allows adequate fluid replacement without forcing an iatrogenic diuresis. Daily serum U&Es should be requested to ensure that the creatinine level is falling. In addition, it is imperative to have hourly monitoring of pulse and blood pressure, twice daily lying and standing blood pressure (a drop indicates hypovolaemic status) as well as daily body weight measurements, to provide objective data regarding overall fluid volume status. The requirement for intravenous fluid support usually lasts for 24–72 hours in POD.

Urological intervention in complex cases

In cases of supra-trigonal obstruction, renal failure will not improve with simple catheterisation. In such cases, a repeat USS, or a CT scan (without intravenous contrast) will be able to delineate persistent hydro-ureteronephrosis (Figure 7.6), and occasionally identify a possible cause, such as pelvic mass or retroperitoneal fibrosis. In such cases, which are by definition complex, decompression of the urinary tract has to be performed with percutaneous nephrostomy insertion, to reverse the renal failure.

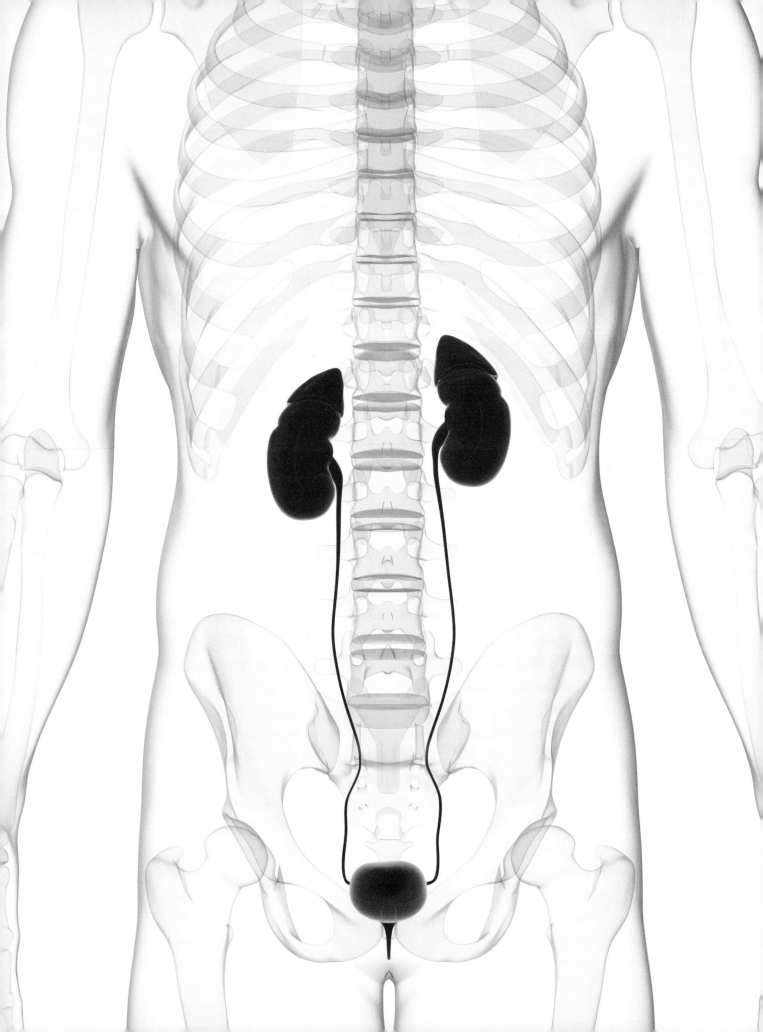

Bladder

Part 3

Chapters

8 Lower urinary tract symptoms

Figure 8.1 Hald diagram showing the relationship between LUTS, BOO and BPE. The intersections of all three are those patients with symptomatic BPE
Source: Hald T *et al. Proceedings of the 4th International Consultation on Benign Prostatic Hyperplasia, Paris, 1997.* SCI, 1993, 129-178.

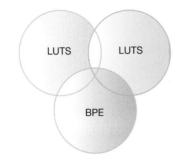

Table 8.1 Symptoms categorisation

Storage symptoms	Voiding symptoms	Post-micturition symptoms
Frequency	Hesitancy	Post-micturition dribbling
Nocturia	Intermittency	Feeling of incomplete bladder emptying
Urgency	Poor stream	
Incontinence	Straining	
	Terminal dribbling	
	Splitting/spraying	

Table 8.2 Frequency volume chart (NB: this is continued for a 24 hour period, over three consecutive days)

Time	Input	Output	Incontinence Yes or No
06:00 am			
07:00 am			

Figure 8.2 Cross-section of the male bladder, prostate and urethra. Disease or dysfunctions in any of these cause LUTS

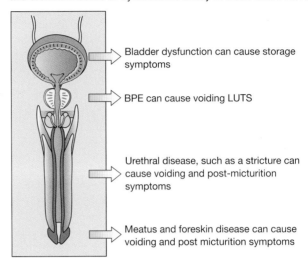

Bladder dysfunction can cause storage symptoms

BPE can cause voiding LUTS

Urethral disease, such as a stricture can cause voiding and post-micturition symptoms

Meatus and foreskin disease can cause voiding and post micturition symptoms

Figure 8.2 McNeal's Zones

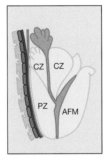

The **transition zone (TZ)**, is the area around the urethra and accounts for 2% of glandular tissue of the normal prostate, The **central zone (CZ)**, is the area around the ejaculatory ducts. The **peripheral zone (PZ)**, encloses the central and trasition zones posteriorly and laterally. Importantly, benign growth of the prostese occurs predominantly in the TZ where as 75% of the prostate cancers occur within The PZ of the prostate. The **anterior fibromuscular stroma zone (AZ)** is on the anterior aspect of the prostate

Table 8.3 Overall management of LUTS in men
Source: NICE guidelines (2010) The management of lower urinary tract symptoms in men

Symptoms/diagnosis	Symptoms/diagnosis
Moderate/severe LUTS	Offer an alpha blocker
OAB	Offer an antichoinergic
UTS and prostate volume >30g, or a PSA >1.4ng/mL (high risk of progression)	Offer a 5ARI
Bathersome moderate to severe LUTS + prostate volume >30g or a PSA >1.4ng/mL	5ARI + alpha blocker
Storage symptoms when alpha blockers fall	Offer an anticholinergic

Lower urinary tract symptoms (LUTS) are a group of symptoms, which were previously referred to as 'prostatism'. The term LUTS recognises the fact that these symptoms occur in both sexes and are not necessarily caused by the prostate. Using the correct terminology is important as not all cases of LUTS are caused by bladder outflow obstruction (BOO) and not all causes of BOO are caused by benign prostatic hyperplasia (BPH) (Figure 8.1). We can broadly categories LUTS into **storage, voiding** and/or **post-micturition** symptoms (Table 8.1). This categorisation helps define the source of the problem (Figure 8.2).

Lower urinary tract symptoms in male patients

Anatomy and pathophysiology

The anatomy of the male lower urinary tract consists of the bladder, prostate, urethra and sphincters. Abnormalities of any of these can cause LUTS in men.

The incidence and propensity to develop BPH increases with age. In the natural history of BPH there is an increase in the normal stromal : epithelial ratio.

BPH represents one of the main causes of male LUTS in men over 50, and can cause acute urinary retention (AUR). The anatomy of the prostate has been described in many different ways; cystoscopically it is often described as having a median lobe and two lateral lobes. More commonly, urologists refer to McNeal's zones when referring to prostate anatomy (Figure 8.3).

Definitions

To help with the history, we have to be able to understand certain urology terms. The International Continence Society (ICS) defines the following terms:

• *Urgency:* the complaint of a sudden compelling desire to pass urine, which is difficult to defer.
• *Frequency:* a complaint by the patient who considers that he/she voids too often by day.
• *Urgency incontinence:* complaint of involuntary leakage accompanied by or immediately preceded by urgency.
• *Weak/intermittent stream:* the patient's perception of reduced urine flow; this flow may even stop and start. This is compared to previous performance or in comparison to others.
• *Hesitancy:* difficulty in initiating micturition resulting in a delay in the onset of voiding after the individual is ready to pass urine.
• *Straining:* the muscular effort used to either initiate, maintain or improve the urinary stream.
• *Terminal dribbling:* when an individual describes a prolonged final part of micturition, when the flow has slowed to a trickle/dribble.
• *Post-micturition dribbling:* where an individual describes the involuntary loss of urine immediately after he or she has finished passing urine, usually after leaving the toilet in men, or after rising from the toilet in women.
• *Incomplete bladder emptying:* a self-explanatory term for a feeling experienced by the individual after passing urine.

• *Acute urinary retention:* a painful, palpable or percussable bladder, when the patient is unable to pass urine.
• *Nocturnal enuresis:* loss of urine occurring during sleep.

Differential diagnosis

Always ensure you rule out alternative causes for LUTS as shown in Box 8.1.

Box 8.1 Causes of lower urinary tract symptoms

• Bladder outflow obstruction
• Overactive bladder syndrome (OAB)/detrusor overactivity
• Combination of bladder outflow obstruction and OAB/detrusor overactivity
• Bladder cancer
• Prostate cancer (men only)
• Stones
• Infection
• Neurological causes
• Nocturnal enuresis
• Excess fluid intake

History and examination

Armed with this knowledge we can perform a focused urological assessment.

Focused history

• *Age* Overall, this is an important risk factor. As the age increases, the risk of developing AUR increases.
• *Predominant symptoms* (Figure 8.1) It is important to establish the predominant symptoms as this can guide initial treatment.
• *Red flags* Nocturnal enuresis, haematuria (think cancer!), bladder pain, neurological symptoms.
• *Previous surgery* For example, transurethral resection of the prostate (TURP), abdominal perineal resection (APR) and spinal surgery leading to a neuropathic bladder. Previous surgery requiring catheterisation.
• *Co-morbidities* Assess fitness for surgery. Parkinson's disease, diabetes and cardiac failure.
• *Drug history* Diuretics, antidepressants, anticholinergic, sympathomimetic, alpha-blockers, 5-alpha reductase inhibitors (5ARIs). These medications can affect bladder and prostate function.

Focused examination

• *Abdominal* Can you feel a palpable bladder?
• *External genitalia* Ensure no phimosis or meatal stenosis.
• *Digital rectal examination (DRE).*
• *Prostate character* Is this benign or malignant feeling?
• *Prostate volume >30 g* Large, medium or small. The bigger the size of the prostate, the higher the chances of developing retention. The prostate volume is very difficult to measure by DRE. However, it is much more accurately measured through a TRUS-guided probe.
• *Anal tone and sensation* If a neurological cause is suspected, this could be an indication of cord compression.
• *Focused neurological examination* Some patients with AUR present with spinal cord compression or cauda equina syndrome.

Basic investigations

Urine dipstick test to check for blood (requires urgent investigation), protein, leucocytes and nitrates (can indicate infection as a cause of symptoms) and glucose.

Midstream urine (MSU) sent for microscopy, culture and sensitivity (MC&S) if urinalysis shows an abnormality.

Frequency/volume chart or bladder diary. This is a record of the volumes voided and the times of micturition over a 24-hour period. Ideally, this should be performed over **three** consecutive days.

International Prostate Symptom Score (IPSS) is an eight-item questionnaire consisting of seven symptom questions and one quality of life (QoL) question.

Or the **International Consultation on Incontinence Questionnaire (ICIQ-MLUTS):** this contains 13 items with subscales for nocturia and OAB and is available in 17 languages. IPSS score of:

0–7 refers to mild symptoms
8–19 refers to moderate symptoms
20–35 refers to severe symptoms.

The higher the IPSS score, the higher the chances of developing AUR.

Blood tests

• *Prostate-specific antigen >1.4 ng/mL:* as PSA is prostate-specific rather than cancer-specific, it can be elevated for a number of reasons. This includes BPE, and therefore as the size of the prostate increases the PSA increases. Strong evidence exists that baseline PSA predicts future prostate growth and that those with elevated PSA levels are at higher risk of developing episodes of AUR and the subsequent need for operative intervention.
• *Glucose:* diabetes can cause polyuria. Patients can present with frequency and nocturia.
• *U&Es:* checking for renal impairment. This is a surrogate marker of upper tract dysfunction.

The NICE guidelines of 2010 suggest onward referral to a **specialist centre** for further urological investigation if patients have:
• **Bothersome** LUTS that have not responded to conservative or drug treatment
• LUTS complicated by renal impairment, retention, urinary tract infection or urological cancer.

Specialised urological investigations

In addition to the basic investigations, once the patient has been referred to the urology clinic we perform the following investigations.

Flow rate and post-void residual ultrasound

This is a non-invasive way of assessing the patient's flow but it **does not give a definitive diagnosis of obstruction, and sometimes further investigations are needed (e.g. urodynamics).**

Some men with a maximum flow rate (Qmax >15 mL/s) can still have obstruction, while those with a low flow can have an underactive detrusor rather than obstruction.

Following this investigation, we can then scan the bladder using ultrasound to assess how much urine is left behind.

Invasive urodynamic investigation

This is a study to assess how the bladder and urethra perform the task of storage and voiding by measuring the pressure inside the bladder. It is an invasive test but is the definitive method to establish a functional diagnosis for the patient's symptoms. This is reserved for:
• Younger men <50 years
• Equivocal flow rates:
  • Elderly patients
  • Flow rates >15 mL/s
  • Very low flow and suspected bladder failure
• Patients with neurological symptoms or after major pelvic surgery
• Previous unsuccessful invasive treatment
• Severe storage symptoms.

Ultrasound renal tract

NICE guidelines, 2010, suggest an ultrasound of the renal tract in the following situations:
• Chronic retention
• Haematuria
• Sterile pyruria
• Recurrent urinary tract infection
• Profound symptoms and pain.

Long-term sequelae of benign prostatic obstruction

• Symptomatic progression
• AUR
• UTI
• Bladder calculi
• Renal insufficiency
• Incontinence
• Haematuria.

Management

1 Conservative (observation only)
2 Medical management:
  • Alpha-adrenoreceptor blockers
  • 5ARI
  • Anticholinergic receptor blockers
  • Beta 3 agonists
  • Phosphodiesterase type 5 (PDE5) inhibitors
3 Surgical therapy.

Conservative

This is suitable for patients with mild–moderate symptoms with a mild *bother* score. Lifestyle changes are important (e.g. reduced caffeine and fluid), bladder retraining exercises and treating constipation.

Not all patients with LUTS need treatment and a significant proportion will either improve or remain stable symptomatically. Some will get better with simply lifestyle modification advice.

Medical management

Alpha-adrenoreceptor blockers are thought to reduce the dynamic effect of obstruction by causing smooth muscle relaxation of the bladder neck. Their side effects are mainly postural hypotension and retrograde ejaculation, but they can also cause erectile dysfunction and floppy iris syndrome.

5ARI (type 2 5ARI is the dominant isoform): finasteride is a type 2 5ARI that reduces prostate volume, improves IPSS score and furthermore increases urinary flow to some degree. In this regard, it prevents the progression of BPH-related symptoms. However, finasteride can take at least 6 months to improve symptoms. It has the effect of reducing total PSA by 50%. Its adverse effects include reduced libido, breast symptoms, reduced ejaculatory volume and erectile dysfunction. Dutasteride is a both a combined type 1 and 2 5ARI. It has been reported to have a quicker onset of symptom improvement in those patients with larger prostates and therefore may be considered in those patients with large prostates with severe bothersome symptoms.

The rationale behind **combination therapy** (combined alpha-blocker and 5ARI) is that it has a quicker onset of symptom relief than either alpha-blocker or 5ARI alone; furthermore, it reduces clinical progression. This is the treatment of choice for moderate to severe LUTS where the prostate volume is >30 g or the PSA is >1.4 ng/mL.

Anticholinergic receptor blockers (antimuscarinics) can be used in patients where storage symptoms predominate.

Muscarinic receptors are present on many epithelial cell surfaces including the urothelial cells. There are five muscarinic receptor subtypes (M1–M5). The M2 and M3 receptor type are mainly expressed within the bladder.

Frequency, urgency and nocturia form the overactive bladder syndrome and can be caused by detrusor overactivity (urodynamic diagnosis). In men, detrusor overactivity can be the primary cause of storage symptoms or be secondary to bladder outflow obstruction. Inhibiting these contractions with (M2 and M3) antagonists (referred to as anticholinergics) can lead to fewer storage symptoms.

Although you may think that prescribing medications that relax the detrusor muscle would lead to a high rate of urinary retention in men with bladder outflow obstruction, it is not the case. Through systematic review and meta-analysis, NICE currently recommend oxybutynin or tolterodine immediate release as first-line anticholinergics but these drugs are less selective and therefore can have a high side effect profile. NICE do not recommend giving oxybutynin to the elderly. If these anticholinergics are not tolerated or efficacious then alternative newer, more selective, modified release anticholinergics can be used (Table 8.3).

Beta 3 adrenoceptor agonists. Recently, a drug with a new mechanism of action for treating overactive bladder syndrome has been developed. Mirabegron binds to the beta 3 receptor found in the bladder leading to smooth muscle relaxation. NICE recommend its use in those patients in whom 'anticholinergics are contraindicated or clinically ineffective, or have unacceptable side effects'.

PDE5 inhibitors are thought to increase intracellular cyclic guanosine monophosphate, thereby relaxing the smooth muscle tone of the prostate, bladder and urethra.

Surgical management

The following are commonly deemed indications for surgical intervention:

1 Recurrent urinary tract infections
2 Recurrent or refractory bouts of urinary retention
3 Bladder stones
4 Haematuria that does not settle with 5ARIs
5 Elevated creatinine due to BOO
6 Worsening symptoms despite maximum medical therapy.

TURP is the most common operation for benign prostatic obstruction (BPO); traditionally a monopolar resection in the UK, although some centres perform biopolar resections.

Lasers have also been used to unblock the prostatic obstruction. The holmium:yttrium-aluminium-garnet (Ho:YAG) laser (wavelength 2140 nm) is a pulsed solid-state laser that is absorbed by water. Coagulation and necrosis are limited to 3–4 mm, which is enough to obtain adequate haemostasis. Holmium laser enucleation of the prostate (HoLEP) results in laser resection of the prostate and relief of LUTS, with long-term functional results comparable to TURP and open prostatectomy. It is often used for large prostate resections. NICE recommend that HoLEP procedures should be performed in specialists centres.

Green light laser: the kalium-titanyl-phosphate (KTP) and the lithium triborate (LBO) lasers both work at a wavelength of 532 nm. Their energy is absorbed by haemoglobin but not by water. Vaporisation leads to removal of prostatic tissue and hence relief of BPO, and the subsequent reduction of LUTS. This procedure is often used in those patients who are anticoagulated or have multiple cardiovascular comorbidities.

NICE have also recently recommended the Urolift procedure. This is a minimally invasive procedure with a better side effect profile. However, symptom scores reduce on average by 50% but it is a relatively new procedure.

Open operations to remove the benign prostate are very rarely performed in the UK.

Lower urinary tract symptoms in female patients

The anatomy of the female lower urinary tract comprises the bladder, the external urethral sphincter and the urethra. The female urethra (4 cm) is much shorter than that of males (about 22 cm).

Four main factors contribute to normal female bladder function and continence:

1 Bladder compliance
2 Efficient urethral sphincter
3 Efficient urethral support
4 Adequate urethral mucosal coaptation.

As in men, LUTS in females are broadly categorised into storage, voiding and post-micturition symptoms.

Storage symptoms include frequency, urgency, nocturia, **pain** and **incontinence**. Voiding and post-micturition symptoms are experienced in the voiding phase.

Differential diagnosis

There are many non-functional causes of female LUTS that need to be excluded before attributing the symptoms to idiopathic LUTS (Table 8.2).

Differential diagnosis in those presenting with storage symptoms

- Frequency of urination and nocturia:
  - Polyuria
  - Detrusor overactivity
  - Low bladder compliance.
- Urgency/urgency incontinence:
  - Sensory urgency
  - Overactive bladder syndrome
  - Low bladder compliance.
- Post-void dribble:
  - Urethral diverticulum
  - Urethral obstruction
  - Vaginal pooling.

Differential diagnosis in those presenting with voiding symptoms

- Urethral obstruction
- Voiding at low volumes
- Detrusor underactivity
- Detrusor sphincter dyssynergia (DSD): this is an urodynamic diagnosis characterised by increased sphincter contraction in conjunction with involuntary detrusor contractions. DSD typically occurs in those with a supra-sacral spinal cord lesion, and can lead to AUR, renal failure and bladder stone formation.

Overactive bladder syndrome

The ICS defines OAB as 'urgency, usually with urinary frequency and nocturia, with or without urgency urinary incontinence'. This is based on the assumption that there is no urinary infection or other obvious aetiology. Therefore OAB syndrome is a term based on symptom presentation. **Detrusor overactivity** can only be diagnosed on urodynamics and is defined as the presence of involuntary detrusor contractions during filling cystometry, which can be spontaneous or provoked.

History and examination

Focused history

- Age
- Fluid intake: including volume and type (caffeinated, carbonated, alcoholic drinks).

Storage symptoms: Try to establish the predominant type of symptoms:
- *Urgency:* it is important to note how long the patient can postpone her desire to void after she gets the 'strong urge/desire to void'.
- Frequency

- *Urgency incontinence:* does she leak with the urgency or with exercise/effort (called stress urinary incontinence)? If so, how many pads does she use?
- *Nocturia:* does she wake to pass urine after she has gone to sleep?
- *Pain:* some patients experience suprapubic, urethral or vaginal pain and discomfort. Try to establish if there are precipitating or relieving features. In particular, is the pain worse with a full bladder and relieved by voiding?

Voiding symptoms

- Weak/intermittent stream
- Straining
- Hesitancy
- Incomplete emptying
- Terminal dribbling
- Dysuria (exclude infection)
- *Post-micturition:* post-micturition dribbling
- *Previous surgery:* ask about previous obstetric and gynaecological procedures, abdomino-perineal resections and previous radiotherapy. How many vaginal deliveries?
- *Co-morbidities:* assess fitness for surgery. Certain neurological diseases are known to affect the bladder and sphincter (multiple sclerosis, spinal cord or lumbar disc disease, myelodysplasia, Parkinson's disease and multi-system atrophy). Does the patient have a raised BMI measured as weight (kg)/height^2 (m^2)?
- *Drug history:* tricyclic antidepressants, alpha-adrenergic agonists and parasympathomimethics can affect bladder function.
- *Social history:* smoker or any occupational exposure to carcinogens?

Focused examination

The patient's abdomen should be examined to check for masses, hernias or a distended bladder. A pelvic examination (i.e. a vaginal examination) should be performed:
- To assess the oestrogen status of the vagina
- To check for pelvic floor muscle contraction
- To check for a pelvic mass
- To perform a cough provocation test: does she leak on coughing?

Using a Sims' speculum, the anterior and posterior vaginal compartments can be examined in the lateral position to check for prolapse.

A focused neurological examination should be carried out, if necessary, to check for the afferent (perineal sensation) and motor distributions (S3 dermatome by asking the patient to spread their toes).

Basic investigations

Following the history and examination a **urine dipstick** test should be performed (recurrent UTIs and haematuria in women over 40 suggests an urgent referral to a urologist according to NICE guidelines). A **three-day bladder diary** documents the type and volume of fluid intake, frequency, voided volumes, incontinence episodes and the number of pads used.

Specialised urological investigations

1 Perform a **validated questionnaire** to assess the impact of the patient's symptoms on their QoL: such as the **Kings Health Questionnaire** or **ICIQ-Female Lower Urinary Tract Symptoms questionnaire (ICIQ-FLUTS)**.

2 Flow rate and examination of the post-void residual urinary volume.

3 Current NICE guidelines do not recommend performing a routine cystoscopic examination of the patient's bladder as part of the initial assessment. However, if patients also have suprapubic pain or haematuria this examination would be appropriate.

4 Urodynamic investigation: NICE guidelines recommend urodynamics only after conservative treatments have failed and invasive therapy is being considered. Urodynamics is recommended before surgery in all women who have:

- Symptoms of OAB leading to a clinical suspicion of detrusor overactivity
- Symptoms suggestive of voiding dysfunction or anterior compartment prolapse
- Previous surgery for stress incontinence.

 It should also be considered:

- When the other diagnostic tests have been inconclusive
- When major radical pelvic surgery has been performed
- When suspected neurological pathologies that affect the bladder and sphincter are known to be involved (e.g. Parkinson's disease, multiple sclerosis, spinal cord injury amongst many others).

Management

1 Conservative management and lifestyle modifications
2 Bladder training
3 Medical management
4 Botulinum toxin intravesical injections
5 Surgery: sacral nerve stimulation, clam ileocystoplasty or ileal conduit urinary diversion.

Conservative management and lifestyle modifications

NICE recommend first-line treatment for LUTS in female patients to be lifestyle interventions including:
- Caffeine reduction
- Modification of fluid intake
- Weight lose in women with a BMI of >30.

 If the patient has stress or mixed incontinence, then supervised pelvic floor muscle training of at least 3 months' duration should be given.

 If the symptoms are predominantly storage, then bladder training has been shown to be more effective than controls in randomised control trials. If patients do not achieve satisfactory benefit with bladder training programs alone then consider a combination of drug treatment with bladder training.

Drug therapy

In postmenopausal women with signs of vaginal atrophy and symptoms of OAB, NICE recommend topical vaginal oestrogen therapy.

Anticholinergics have been covered in the section on LUTS in male patients. In men we often try to establish if there is concomitant bladder outflow obstruction whereas in women it is important to establish if symptoms are predominantly overactive or stress/effort related.

The efficacy, mode of action and use of **anticholinergic receptor blockers** has been discussed and they are used similarly (perhaps more so) in females to establish the desired effect.

Desmopressin is highly effective in the treatment of nocturia, especially if the patient has nocturnal polyuria. The main side effect of note is that of a dilutional hyponatraemia in approximately 10% of patients and therefore sodium levels need to be monitored.

Surgical management

The surgical management of female urinary incontinence is covered in Chapter 9. However, the placement of botulinum toxin A intravesically can be given as an outpatient local anaesthetic procedure for those with OAB. Although the main proposed mechanism of action is that Botox binds to the presynaptic nerve terminals leading to the inhibition of acetylcholine, there are many other afferent and efferent possible effects. Overall, the efficacy is very good in idiopathic or neurogenic detrusor overactivity, but patients need to be counselled carefully as the effects are temporary, requiring repeat injections and 10–20% of patients need to perform intermittent self-catheterisation as a result of retention.

Other treatments include sacral nerve stimulation, clam ileocystoplasty and even urinary diversion in severe cases.

Urinary retention

The retention of urine can be acute or chronic.

Acute urinary retention

Acute urinary retention (AUR) is defined is a painful inability to pass urine, with subsequent relief by immediate catheterisation and bladder drainage.

 It is imperative to document:
- The size of the catheter
- The type of catheter: two or three-way, long-term or short-term or even a suprapubic catheter and so on
- Balloon volume
- **Residual urine volume.**

 If the residual is <300 mL, urologists often question the diagnosis of AUR. In general, residuals need to be <20% of the functional bladder capacity. So if the bladder capacity is 500 mL, then a residual of <100 mL is acceptable. Typically, if the residual volume is >800 mL, this is often referred to as **acute on chronic retention.** Residuals of >1.5 L are usually regarded as **chronic retention.**

Pathology

Overall, there are four mechanisms that lead to urinary retention:
1 High resistance in the urethra (BOO)
2 Low bladder pressure (impaired bladder contractility)

3 Impaired sensory or motor supply to the bladder

4 Impaired coordination between bladder contraction the subsequent relaxation of the external sphincter.

In men, a high IPSS score, large prostate volumes, a low Q_{max}, advancing age and previous episodes of retention are all strong risk predictors for AUR.

Causes in men and women

1 Spontaneous (i.e. there is no cause!)

2 Precipitating causes:
  • Drug-induced: anticholinergics, anaesthetic agents epidural and spinal anaesthesia
  • Bleeding: clots
  • Pain postoperatively
  • Neurological injury: multiple sclerosis; S2–4 compression/injury, damage to dorsal columns, suprasacral spinal cord injury, cauda equina
  • Fracture: pelvis causing urethral injury
  • Surgery: radical pelvic surgery damaging parasympathetic plexus, post surgery for stress incontinence
  • Gynaecological: pelvic prolapse
  • Malignancy: prostate, pelvic mass
  • Benign prostatic enlargement
  • Constipation especially in the elderly
  • Infection.

Management

A history and examination (including lower limb neurological examination if appropriate) is performed. The following points can be considered as initial management:
  • DRE/pelvic examination in a female
  • FBC, U&Es and estimated glomerular filtration rate (eGFR)
  • Immediate catheterisation and recording the residual
  • Urine dipstick.

Your subsequent management is individualised, specific and tailored to the patient, especially if retention is spontaneous.

Causes in men

If there is a precipitating event one must treat the cause and then perform a trial without catheterisation (TWOC), if this is deemed appropriate. If these causes have been excluded, a TWOC could be performed with the addition of an alpha-adrenoreceptor blocker (e.g. tamsulosin 400 µg once daily). This is typically given for 24–48 hours prior to removing the catheter. It can then be continued if needed depending on the patient's LUTS prior to the episode of AUR.

Alternatively, one could try a prostate shrinking drug (5ARIs) with or without alpha-adrenoreceptor blocker for a few months then perform a TWOC. 5ARIs reduce the risk of AUR episodes and the need for BPO-related surgery.

A failure to void despite excluding precipitating causes and the initiating of medical therapy indicates the need for surgery in the form of a TURP, in those who are surgically fit.

In those with significant co-morbidity or those not wishing to have surgical intervention, bladder drainage can be performed in the form of clean intermittent self-catheterisation (CISC) or a long-term catheter (LTC). Importantly, these patients need to counselled appropriately about the risks, benefits and complications, with the relevant specialist nurse and district nurse involvement throughout their care.

Causes in women

A TWOC is performed once precipitating causes have been treated and excluded. If they fail to void, CISC or LTC is performed until normal voiding returns.

Chronic retention

Anyone who leaves a residual volume of urine after voiding can be said to have chronic retention. Presentation is typically painless with the patient not knowing that they have retention.

Importantly, chronic retention can be:
• **Low pressure:** no hydronephrosis, normal creatinine
• **High pressure:** raised creatinine, which typically improves following catheterisation. There is often hydronephrosis.

However, **acute on chronic retention** is often described as the painful inability to void with residuals of >800 mL. Again, this can be a low or a high-pressure system.

In a low-pressure system, the upper tracts are 'safe'; there is typically no deterioration in renal function. The patient voids, but there is still a significant residual volume of urine within the bladder but this will not cause any significant impairment to the upper tracts or renal function.

If there are no bothersome LUTS, UTI or upper tract compromise, we can monitor the residual volumes, keeping a close eye on the renal function and upper tracts (via a renal ultrasound scan). Therefore no treatment is absolutely necessary; however, we could consider a TURP if the patient develops bothersome LUTS or UTI in a low-pressure system.

High pressure chronic retention

The concepts and management of high pressure chronic retention (HPCR) are of paramount importance in urological practice.

There is often a long history of **urinary leakage** but only at night when the patient is asleep (nocturnal enuresis). You may visually see a **grossly distended bladder**. Residual volumes are typically >800 mL and classically the **end voided detrusor pressure** is thought to be >30 cmH$_2$O on urodynamics.

There is typically **renal dysfunction**, with concomitant **bilateral hydro-ureteronephrosis.** Once the catheter is inserted, the residual can be large, but renal function normally improves over time. It is imperative to correct any electrolyte disturbance to prevent cardiac dysrhythmias. The patient may have **significant diuresis (>200 mL/hour for 6 consecutive hours)** following bladder drainage and managing this is very important. A diuresis occurs for the following reasons:
• *Physiological:* excretion of retained fluid and electrolytes
• *Pathological:* decreased response to collecting ducts to antidiuretic hormone (ADH):
  • Increased production atrial natriuretic peptide (ANP)
  • Loss of corticomedullary concentration gradient
  • Osmotic diuresis due to increased urea excretion.

Initial management

These patients typically require admission to hospital.

• Insert catheter and record the post-void residual as described earlier
• U&Es initially and daily
• Daily weights
• Lying and standing blood pressure to look for a symptomatic postural drop of 20 mmHg
• Hourly urine output
• Although initially the diuresis is physiological, intravenous fluids may be required if the diuresis persists and becomes pathological or the patient develops symptoms.

The patient can develop post-decompression haematuria; slow decompression is no longer recommended and the haematuria normally settles in 48–72 hours.

Subsequent management

• Renal tract ultrasound to look for **bilateral hydro-ureteronephrosis and substance of the renal parenchyma.** The hydro-ureteronephrosis usually settles with bladder drainage and as renal function improves.
• TWOC and medical management are ***not* appropriate** in the management of these patients as these will lead to renal failure and significant upper tract dilatation.
• TURP or LTC/CISC are the mainstay of treatment in the management of HPCR.

Further reading

Abrams P, Cardozo L, Fall M, *et al*; Standardisation Sub-Committee of the International Continence Society. The standardisation of terminology in lower urinary tract function: report from the standardisation sub-committee of the International Continence Society. *Urology* 2003; 61: 37–49.

European Association of Urology (EAU). EAU Guidelines on the assessment of non-neurogenic male lower urinary tract symptoms including benign prostatic obstruction. *Eur Urol* 2015; 67: 1099–1109.

Hald T, *et al. Proceedings of the 4th International Consultation on Benign Prostatic Hyperplasia, Paris, 1997.* SCI; 1993: 129–178.

McNeal JE. The zonal anatomy of the prostate. *Prostate* 1981; 2: 35–49.

NICE Guidelines. *Lower urinary tract symptoms in men: management.* May 2010. https://www.nice.org.uk/guidance/cg97 (accessed 18 July 2016).

NICE Guidelines. *Urinary incontinence in women: management.* September 2013. https://www.nice.org.uk/guidance/cg171 (accessed 18 July 2016).

NICE Pathways. *Overactive bladder drugs.* September 2014. http://pathways.nice.org.uk/pathways/urinary-incontinence-in-women#path=view%3A/pathways/urinary-incontinence-in-women/overactive-bladder-drugs.xml&content=view-index (accessed 18 July 2016).

9 Urinary tract infections

Table 9.1 Factors that affect the risk of urinary tract infection (UTI)

Increased risk	Reduced risk
• Renal obstruction • Vesicoureteric reflux • Pregnancy • Spinal cord injuries • High urinary glucose (diabetes) • Use of antibiotics • Menopause • Benign prostatic hyperplasia • Genetic predisposition • Immunocompromise (e.g. HIV)	• Urinary pH 5.5–6.5 • High urinary urea concentration • *Staphylococci* • *Streptococci* • *Lactobacilli* • Antegrade flow in urethra

Table 9.2 Common bacterial causes of UTI

Common urinary oathogens (Gram-negative unless specified)
Community acquired • *Escheerichia coli* • *Klebsiella* • *Proteus* • *Enterococcus faecalis* (Gram-positive) **Hospital acquired (in addition to above)** • *Pseudomonas aeruginosa* • *Citrobacter* • *Serratia* **Catheter associated** • *Gardenerella vaginalis* • Mycoplasma (derived from Gram-positive, but test negative as lack cell wall) • *Ureaplasma urealyticum* (derived from Gram-positive, but test negative as lack cell wall)

Figure 9.1 Gram-positive *Staphylococcus aureus*
Source: Patho, http://commons.wikimedia.org/wiki/File: Purulent_inflammation,_Gram_stain_3.jpg. Used under CC-BY-SA 3.0

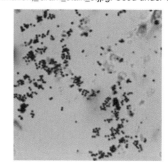

Figure 9.2 Gram-negative rod-shaped *Escherichia coli*.
Source: Bobjgalindo, http://commons.wikimedia.org/wiki/ File:E_choli_Gram.JPG. Used under CC-BY-SA 3.0

Figure 9.3 Antibiotic sensitivity testing.
Source: Dr Graham Beards, http://commons.wikimedia.org/wiki/ File:M._cat_BSAC.JPG. Used under CC-BY-SA 3.0

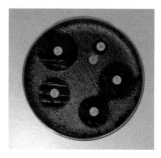

Pathophysiology of urinary tract infection

Definitions

A **urinary tract infection** (UTI) is the inflammation of the lining of the urinary tract in response to invasion by a pathogen, most commonly associated with the presence of bacteria and white blood cells (WBCs) in the urine. This is in contrast to **bacteriuria** and **pyuria**, which describe merely the presence of bacteria and WBCs respectively, and do not necessarily indicate an active infection. Bacteriuria alone can be the result of sample contamination from skin flora or colonisation of an indwelling catheter. Sterile pyuria in the absence of antibiotic treatment warrants investigation for stone disease, urinary tract malignancy and tuberculosis.

The urinary tract is usually sterile. Bacteria enter the urinary tract by **ascending** from the anus to the urethra and then into the bladder. Although bacteria can spread in the blood (haematogenous route) or through lymphatic channels (lymphatic route), these routes are extremely rare. The symptoms of a UTI are called **cystitis**.

Uncomplicated and complicated UTIs

An uncomplicated UTI occurs in an otherwise healthy patient with a structurally and functionally normal urinary tract. An infection can be described as complicated if the patient has any factors that increase the risk of acquiring bacteria and/or decrease the efficacy of antimicrobial therapy. These include any structural or functional abnormality of the urinary tract, immunocompromise of the host and increased virulence or antimicrobial resistance of the pathogen. Most of these patients are children, elderly, pregnant, men, diabetic, immunosuppressed or those with indwelling urinary catheters. Table 9.1 shows factors that increase the risk of UTI and those that are protective.

Common organisms that cause UTIs

Most UTIs are caused by Gram-negative facultative anaerobes originating from bowel flora. *Escherichia coli* is the most common cause of UTIs, accounting for 85% of community-acquired and 50% of hospital-acquired infections. *Staphylococcus epidermidis* and *Candida albicans* originate from the flora of the vagina or perineal skin. Common UTI-causing bacteria are listed in Table 9.2.

Gram staining

A Gram stain is typically the first step in classifying an unknown bacterium (Figures 9.1 and 9.2). It is performed by applying crystal violet to a bacterial smear on a slide for 1–2 minutes. This is then poured off and Gram's iodine added for 1–2 minutes. After this time, the iodine is poured off and the stain decolourised by washing with acetone for 2–3 seconds. The slide is then washed with water and safranin counterstain added for 2 minutes. Finally, the slide is washed with water and dried.

The cell wall of Gram-positive bacteria retains the purple colour of crystal violet because of the presence of much higher concentrations of peptidoglycan, whereas that of Gram-negative bacteria does not and only takes up the pink safranin counterstain.

Urine cultures

Traditionally, a urine sample is processed by centrifuging 5–10 mL of the specimen at 2000 revolutions per minute (r.p.m.) for 5 minutes. The sediment is then mounted on a microscope slide, and examined for red blood cells, white blood cells and bacteria. The number of each cell in a high power field is noted and converted to a number per millilitre. A figure of 10^3 bacteria per mL suggests the presence of an infection.

Samples of 0.1 mL urine are delivered on to each half of a split-agar plate containing blood agar on half for Gram-positive organisms and eosin-methylene blue on the other half for Gram-negative organisms. The number of colonies is then estimated after an overnight incubation. If few or none have grown, the test is reported as negative.

A busy city hospital microbiology department can process over 1000 urine samples every day from its inpatients and surrounding general practices. It is therefore no surprise that the modern microbiology laboratory is highly automated, improving efficiency and allowing for greater resources to be devoted to unusual specimens.

Samples over 2 mL in volume are dispensed into an automated microscopy machine, which centrifuges the urine to separate the cells from the fluid. The sediment is then passed under a high-power digital microscope and multiple images taken and processed digitally to identify key cell types and numbers. Each machine can process up to 80 samples an hour and store the resulting images for future reference.

Identifying bacteria type is expedited by the use of advanced culture media containing colour-changing chromogens that react to specific components of the growing bacteria. Thus, traditional microscopy is rarely required.

Antibiotic sensitivity is assessed by culturing the organism on an agar plate with small discs of paper impregnated with antibiotics commonly used to treat the bacterium cultured. After 24–48 hours the presence or absence of bacterial colonies around each antibiotic is reported as **sensitive, equivocal** or **resistant** (Figure 9.3).

Figure 9.4 Urine dip test showing the presence of leucocytes (top) and blood

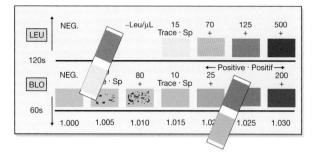

Figure 9.5 An example urine culture report

Microbiology report

Name: Joe Bloggs
DOB: 01/01/1970
Hosp. No: 123456

Specimen: Urine
Direct microscopy: Gram – ve rods
                     WBCs   50-100/cmm
                     RBCs   Scanty
                     Epithelial cells +
Culture: E.coli
                     > 100,000 per mL isolated

Disc sensitivity

Trimethoprim R
Ciprofloxacin S
Amoxicillin R
Gentamicin S
Amikacin S

Table 9.3 Common reactions used in urine dip analysis

Test	Chromogen	Colour change	False positives	False negatives
Haemoglobin	Orthotolidine	Blue	Exercise, bleach, dehydration	Vitamin C
Leucocytes	Catalyses production of violet azole	Violet	Vaginal discharge, formalin	Proteinuria
Nitrites	Greiss reaction	Pink	Contamination	Gram +ve bacteria, pseudomonas, ascorbic acid
pH	Methyl red, bromothymol blue	Orange (acid) blue (alkali)	–	–

Table 9.4 Common antibiotics used to treat UTIs

Agent	Target bacteria	Action	Mode of action	Common side-effects and precautions	Relevance in pregnancy	Dose/timing
Penicillins (e.g. amoxicillin)	Gram +ve	Bactericidal	Interference with bacterial cell wall synthesis	Hypersensitivity, diarrhoea	Safe	TDS 1 g IV/ –250–500mg PO
Cephalosporins (cephalexin)	E. coli Klebsiella Proteus	Bactericidal	Interference with bacterial cell wall synthesis	Hypersensitivity, diarrhoea	Safe	BD –500mg PO
Macrolides (erythromycin)	Chlamydia Syphilis	Bacteriostatic	Inhibition of ribosomal protein synthesis	Diarrhoea and vomiting, arrhythmia, reversible deafness, anaphylaxis	Unsafe: hepatotoxicity and pyloric stenosis	QDS –250–500mg PO
Quinolones (ciprofloxacin)	E. coli Klebsiella Proteus(incl Prostatitis)	Bacteriostatic	Prevention of DNA replication by inhibition of DNA gyrase	Tendon damage (higer risk when given with steroids), diarrhoea, contraindiciated in epileptics, interaction with warfarin	Unsafe	BD –250–500mg PO/IV
Tetracyclines (doxycycline)	Chlamydia	Bacteriostatic	Inhibition of ribosomal protein synthesis	Hepatotoxicity, deposition in growing bones and teeth	Unsafe	OD –100mg PO (2 doses on first day)
Trimethoprim	E. coli Klebsiella Proteus	Bacteriostatic	Prevention of DNA replication by inhibition of dihydrofolate reductase	Thrombocytopenia, artefactual rise in serum creatinine	Unsafe in first trimester	BD –200mg PO
Aminoglycosides (gentamicin)	Pseudomonas Proteus Serratia Staphylococcus	Bactericidal	Inhibition of ribosomal protein synthesis	Nephrotoxicity, ototoxicity, impairs neuromuscular transmission, caution in elderly and renal impairment	Unsafe in second and third trimesters	IM / IV –3–5mg/Kg
Nitrofurantoin	E. coli E. Faecalis Citrobacter	Bactericidal	Damages bacterial DNA by inhibiting multiple enzyme systems	Acute and chronic lung toxicity, hepatotoxicity, allergic reactions, inadequate concentration if GFR<50, nausea and vomiting	Unsafe in third trimester	QDS –50–100mg PO

Investigation and treatment of cystitis

Diagnosis

UTIs can present with dysuria, frequency, urgency, foul-smelling urine and, occasionally, suprapubic pain, haematuria, nausea and vomiting. Particularly in the elderly, symptoms can be absent or non-specific, such as disorientation, confusion and hallucinations.

Urine dip

Urine test strips are thin strips of plastic holding multiple squares of paper impregnated with colour-changing chromogenic reagents to detect various characteristics of the urine. Specific instructions and a comparison chart are supplied by the manufacturer. Generally, the stick is completely immersed in the urine sample and drawn out along the side of the sample pot to remove excess fluid. After a pre-set amount of time (usually 1–5 minutes) the colour of the chromogen is compared with the reference chart (Figure 9.4) to determine the result of the test. Common reagents and false positives are listed in Table 9.3.

For a UTI, the key indicators are nitrites and leucocytes. Bacteria convert nitrates from the urine into nitrites, and leucocytes enter the urine as part of the inflammatory response. The combination of both positive results has a sensitivity (the proportion of positive samples correctly identified as such) of 75–84% and a specificity (the proportion of negative samples correctly identified) of 82–98%.

How to collect a mid-stream urine sample

For women: spread the labia, wash and cleanse the peri-urethral area with a moist gauze from front to back, void the first 100–150 mL urine in the toilet and then place the wide-mouthed sterile container to collect the next 10–15 mL.

For men: retract the foreskin (if uncircumcised), wash the glans penis with soap and rinse with water, keep the foreskin retracted, void the first 100–150 mL urine in the toilet and then place the wide-mouthed sterile container to collect the next 10–15 mL.

Collected samples should be cultured within a few hours or refrigerated immediately and then cultured within 24 hours. Remember to label the container with the patient's details and not only the type of sample but how it was collected – an ascitic tap (urine collected from the suprapubic route by a needle and syringe) and a catheter urine sample can look identical but are interpreted very differently.

Interpreting urine cultures

Figure 9.5 shows an example of a typical urine culture report. It is essential to first check that the sample is from the correct patient and time. If there are no significant quantities of leucocytes, consider that there could be contamination of the sample or colonisation of an indwelling urinary catheter. Always correlate any test result with the clinical status of the patient. If blood is repeatedly present, especially without a convincing infection, investigation for urinary tract malignancy is mandatory. In the case of a confirmed infection, the antibiotic sensitivities can be used to guide treatment choice.

Imaging

UTIs are not diagnosed based upon imaging, but imaging can be valuable in the identification of both causes and serious sequelae of urosepsis.

In the outpatient clinic, urinary flow rate measurement and a post-voiding bladder volume ultrasound can be performed to identify signs of bladder outflow obstruction and incomplete emptying. Flexible cystoscopy can identify causes of obstruction as well as malignancy and calculi within the bladder, but should not be carried out during an acute infection because of the risk of sepsis and inadequate views caused by debris within the bladder.

Ultrasound and CT of the urinary tract can identify upper urinary tract obstruction, collections and malignancy. CT has the benefit of higher resolution, better visualisation of the ureter and greater sensitivity for pathology outside the urinary tract, but is associated with a significant dose of ionising radiation.

Treatment

In the case of a simple UTI demonstrated on urine dip analysis, it is appropriate to prescribe an antibiotic. The choice of antibiotic should be guided by severity of the infection, available culture results and local prescribing protocol which reflect prevalent organisms within the local community. It is always important to consider a patient's co-morbidities and allergies when selecting an appropriate antibiotic. Table 9.4 describes commonly used antimicrobial agents in the context of UTI.

There is a role for long-term low-dose prophylactic antibiotics in patients with recurrent infections when other causes have been excluded. The risk of antibiotic resistance in these circumstances should always be considered.

Prevention

Many UTIs can be prevented by minimising the risk of pathogens entering into and proliferating in the urinary tract. This can be achieved by wiping away from the urethra following defecation, voiding after sexual intercourse and avoiding the use of nylon undergarments. Double-voiding (attempting to empty the bladder twice in quick succession) reduces the amount of stagnant urine within the bladder which can act as a culture medium. Increasing fluid intake is also recommended to reduce urine latency time within the bladder. Avoiding the use of soap and scented shower gel around the urethra also helps to maintain the normal urethral flora, as does the use of topical oestrogen in postmenopausal women. Evidence for the use of cranberry products has been mixed, with some small studies supporting the use of unsweetened cranberry juice or cranberry extract, but meta-analysis unable to demonstrate a clear benefit.

Differential diagnosis

Cystitis is common, but its symptoms are often non-specific. It is therefore important to exclude other possible diagnoses such as:
- Malignancy
- Bladder outflow obstruction
- Idiopathic bladder overactivity
- Renal disease
- Urolithiasis.

Figure 9.6 Complications of UTIs

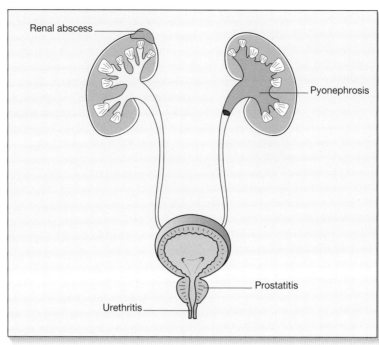

Renal abscess

Pyonephrosis

Prostatitis

Urethritis

Figure 9.7 Schistosoma parasite eggs embedded in human bladder tissue

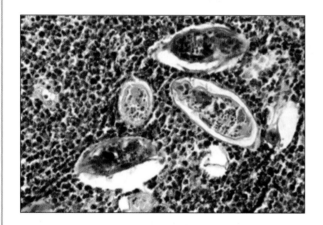

Figure 9.8 Aggressive resection required to manage Fournier's gangrene.
Source: Hayk Margaryan, http://commons.wikimedia.org/wiki/File:Fournier%27s_gangrene_1.jpg. Used under CC-BY-SA 3.0

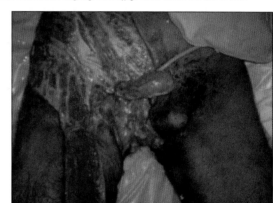

Other infections

While bacterial cystitis is by far the most common UTI, the whole urinary tract can become infected by potentially any pathogen, as shown in Figure 9.6.

Sexually transmitted infections

Sexually transmitted infection (STIs) such as chlamydia and gonorrhoea commonly cause inflammation in the urinary tract, particularly urethritis. However, they can be differentiated from UTIs as they are rarely contracted in situations other than sexual contact and affect locations outside the urinary tract such as the external genitalia and female reproductive tract.

Schistosomiasis (bilharzia)

Schistosomiasis is rarely seen in the western world but is endemic in parts of northern Africa and South America (Figure 9.7). Caused by parasitic water-borne **schistosome** worms with a complex life cycle which includes stages within freshwater snails, the infection most commonly affects the urinary and enteric tracts as well as the liver. Prolonged exposure is a risk factor for the otherwise uncommon squamous cell carcinoma of the bladder.

Prostatitis

Infections of the prostate are caused by the retrograde travel of bacteria from the urinary tract and may or may not be preceded by UTI symptoms. Urine dip tests are frequently unremarkable, but the patient is likely to complain of a chronic perineal pain as well as possible pain on ejaculation and/or haematospermia (blood within the ejaculate). Age distribution is bimodal representing a peak of STIs in early adulthood and outflow obstruction in later life. These are typically treated with doxycycline and ciprofloxacin, respectively, for a minimum of 4 weeks as antibiotic penetration into the prostate is generally poor.

Epididymo-orchitis and Fournier's gangrene

Infections of the testes and epididymi are typically caused in a similar fashion to prostatitis, and take a similarly long time to treat. Patients who are diabetic, alcoholic or malnourished are at greater risk of developing necrotic fasciitis of the perineum, otherwise known as **Fournier's gangrene** (Figure 9.8). Typically, aerobic and anaerobic organisms behave synergistically to create a rapidly spreading gas-forming infection that requires immediate and aggressive tissue debridement to prevent the death of the patient.

Pyelonephritis, pyonephrosis and renal abscess

If a UTI progresses to the kidney, a pyelonephritis can develop. Typically, along with flank pain, such infections cause a much greater degree of fever, rigors, nausea and vomiting, but are usually treated with antibiotics and supportive care. If such an infected upper tract becomes obstructed, a pyonephrosis occurs where the collecting system fills with pus and is unable to drain. Such a situation is an urological emergency and requires immediate decompression with either a nephrostomy or retrograde ureteric stenting.

Severe and recurrent pyelonephritis can also result in a renal or peri-renal abscess. Flank pain, fever, rigors, nausea and vomiting are all common, but other symptoms may be absent as the infection is not necessarily in continuity with the collecting system of the kidney. The presence of an abscess can be confirmed with an ultrasound or contrast-enhanced CT scan. Small abscesses (<3 cm^2) can be treated conservatively, but persistent or larger ones will need image-guided percutaneous drainage.

Further reading

Dalla Palma L, Pozzi-Mucelli F, Ene V. Medical treatment of renal and perirenal abscesses: CT evaluation. *Clin Radiol* 1999; 54: 792–727.

Jepson RG, Williams G, Craig JC. Cranberries for preventing urinary tract infections. *Cochrane Database Syst Rev* 2012; 10: CD001321.

10 Urinary incontinence

Table 10.1 Showing predisposing and exacerbating factors for urinary incontinence

Predisposing	Exacerbating
• Family history • Anatomical pathology (ectopic ureters, fistulae) • Neurological abnormalities (stroke, Parkinson's disease, multiple sclerosis, spinal cord injury) • Pregnancy and childbirth • Pelvic surgeery or radiotherapy	• Older age • Urinary tract infection • Obesity • Respiratory disease or smoking (leading to chronic cough) • Constipation • Menopause • Cognitive impairment

Figure 10.1 Example of a bladder diary

Time	In	Out	Wet	Urgency
	Day 1			
07.00		240mL		
08.00	Orange juice 250mL			
09.00	Coffee 200mL	100mL		✓
10.00		125mL	✓	✓
11.00	Water 400mL			
12.00		100mL		
13.00	Diet Coke 330mL	75mL		✓
14.00				
15.00				
16.00		160mL		
17.00				
18.00	Water 200mL	140mL	✓	✓
19.00		80mL		✓
20.00	Red wine 125mL			
21.00		120mL		
22.00	Water 30mL			
23.00		100mL		
00.00				
01.00				
02.00				
03.00				
04.00		200mL		
05.00				
06.00				

Figure 10.2 Urodynamic system (left) showing urodynamic catheters attached to pressure-transducers. Normal urodynamic trace (right) during bladder, with stable detrusor pressure (Pdet = Pves – Pabd)

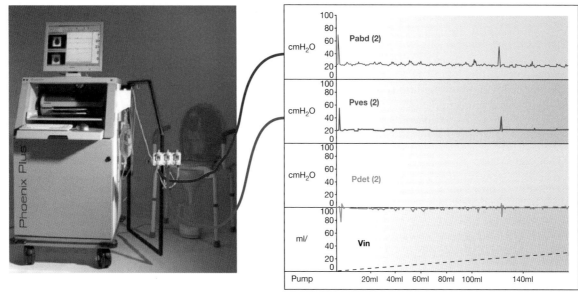

Figure 10.3 Urodynamic trace showing detrusor overactivity. Arrow (⇨) denotes phasic detrusor contractions during bladder filling

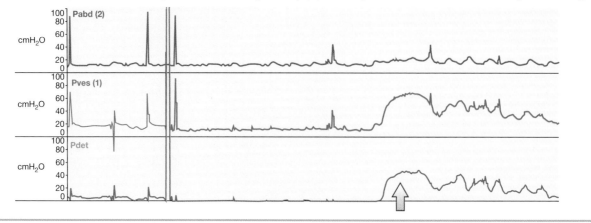

Urology at a Glance, First Edition. Edited by Hashim Hashim and Prokar Dasgupta. © 2017 John Wiley & Sons, Ltd. Published 2017 by John Wiley & Sons, Ltd.
Companion website: www.ataglanceseries.com/urology

Urinary incontinence affects approximately 1 in 12 people, both men and women, of all ages. It can be profoundly debilitating, socially, psychologically, physically and sexually, and is associated with significant costs to individuals and health services.

Definitions

Urinary incontinence is defined by the ICS as the involuntary leakage of urine. It can be further classified according to the situation in which the incontinence occurs.

- **Urgency urinary incontinence (UUI)** is the complaint of involuntary leakage accompanied by or immediately preceded by **urgency** (the sudden compelling desire to pass urine which is difficult to defer). This is a key symptom of overactive bladder syndrome.
- **Overactive bladder (OAB)** is defined by the symptom of urgency with or without urge incontinence, usually with frequency and nocturia. It can occur as a result of a neurological condition (neurogenic) or without an identifiable cause (idiopathic).
- **Stress urinary incontinence (SUI)** is the complaint of involuntary leakage on effort or exertion, sneezing or coughing. It is thought to occur as a result of intrinsic sphincter deficiency (ISD) or urethral hypermobility. ISD is a condition in which the urethral sphincter loses its ability to coapt and generate enough pressure to maintain continence. Urethral hypermobility is the result of weakness of the pelvic floor causing the bladder neck and proximal urethra to descend at times of increased intra-abdominal pressure. Under normal circumstances any rise in intra-abdominal pressure is transmitted equally to both the bladder and proximal urethra, resulting in continence. However, with weakness of the pelvic floor, pressure transmission to the proximal urethra is reduced as it descends under the pubic bone, and so bladder pressure is higher than urethral pressure resulting in incontinence.
- **Mixed urinary incontinence (MUI)** is the complaint of involuntary leakage associated with urgency and also with exertion, effort, sneezing or coughing.
- Urinary incontinence as a result of **chronic urinary retention** results in a non-painful bladder which remains palpable or percussible because of high residual volumes after the patient has passed urine.
- **Continuous urinary incontinence** is the complaint of continuous leakage of urine, and is typically related to an underlying anatomical abnormality (e.g. fistula, ectopic ureter).

Evaluation

A thorough history regarding the patient's symptoms is essential in order to determine the type of incontinence, its impact on the patient's quality of life, the likely cause and any co-morbidities that may impact on potential treatment options.

History

The history should ascertain whether the symptoms are predominantly UUI, SUI or MUI, their onset and duration and the presence of any predisposing or exacerbating factors (Table 10.1). UUI can be assessed with a symptom screening questionnaire with bother score (e.g. ICIQ-UI short form), and severity can be assessed by measuring 24-hour pad weights. Symptoms of bowel dysfunction and pelvic organ prolapse often coexist with urinary incontinence. A thorough drug history to identify medications that could impact upon urinary function should be taken, as well as a review of past medical and surgical history which could impact treatment decisions, such as previous pelvic surgery or radiotherapy.

Examination

The patient's BMI should be documented and overweight patients should be advised to lose weight to improve incontinence symptoms.

An abdominal examination to identify a palpable bladder suggestive of chronic urinary retention with overflow incontinence should be followed by a chaperoned examination of the external genitalia. This should be performed in the left lateral position for women, with a Sims' speculum, in order to identify and grade any pelvic organ prolapse, to exclude vaginal masses and to determine pelvic floor strength. State of tissue oestrogenisation and the presence of visible SUI on coughing or Valsalva manoeuvre should also be documented.

A brief neurological examination assessing anal tone and sensation, and lower limb function should also be performed to exclude a neurological lesion.

Investigation

A urinalysis should be performed to exclude urinary infection, and a flow rate and post-void residual urine measurement should be obtained to exclude voiding dysfunction or chronic retention as a cause. In order to be accurately interpretable, the patient should void at least 150 mL urine. All patients should complete a 3-day bladder diary (Figure 10.1). This records the timing of each void, voided volumes, incontinence episodes, pad usage and fluid intake. The bladder diary provides essential information regarding day and night-time frequency, as well as the presence of **polyuria** (production of more than 40 mL/kg body weight of urine in 24 hours in adults) or **nocturnal polyuria** (production of more than 20–33% of total 24-hour urine production at night) which require specific investigation and treatment. Severity of incontinence should be quantified using pad number and weight.

Urodynamics is a test used to measure the pressure–volume relationship of the bladder during filling and voiding (Figure 10.2). It involves the placement of a small-diameter transurethral catheter in order to measure intravesical pressure, and a rectal catheter to measure intra-abdominal pressure. It is important to measure intra-abdominal pressure so that it can be determined whether any rise in detrusor pressure is caused by coughing or straining, or secondary to detrusor overactivity. Detrusor pressure (pdet) is calculated by subtracting the abdominal pressure (pabd) from the intravesical pressure (pves). The presence of involuntary phasic contractions during bladder filling defines **detrusor overactivity** (Figure 10.3).

It should be reserved for patients whose symptoms have not resolved using conservative therapies. Specifically, this investigation should be performed in the following situations:
- Symptoms of OAB
- Symptoms of voiding difficulty, cystocele or those with neurogenic bladder dysfunction
- Prior to invasive surgical treatment
- Failed previous surgical treatment.

Figure 10.4 Mechanism of action of anticholinergic (left) and β-3 agonists (right)

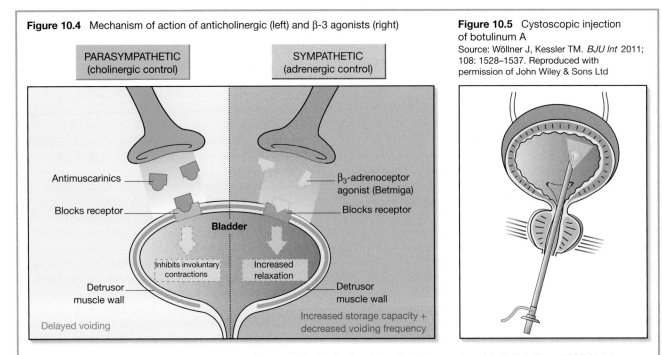

Figure 10.5 Cystoscopic injection of botulinum A

Source: Wöllner J, Kessler TM. *BJU Int* 2011; 108: 1528–1537. Reproduced with permission of John Wiley & Sons Ltd

Figure 10.6 Sacral neuromodulation implant

Source: Wöllner J, Hampel C, Kessler TM. *BJU Int* 2012; 110: 146–159. Reproduced with permission of John Wiley & Sons Ltd

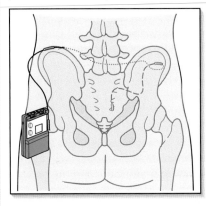

Figure 10.7 Synthetic mid-urethral tapes-retropubic TVT (left) and TOT (right)

Retropubic route

Transobturator route

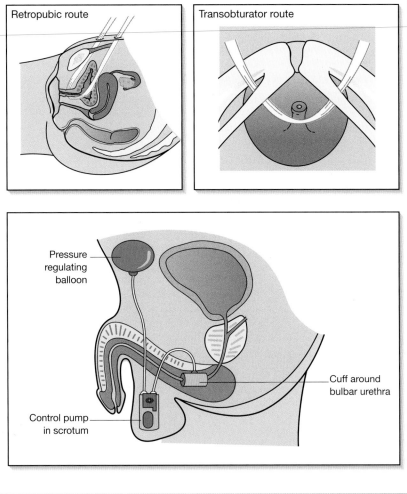

Figure 10.8 The artificial urinary sphincter demonstrating the position of the 3 components: the pressure-regulating balloon in the retro-peritoneal space, the urethral cuff, and the control pump

Pressure regulating balloon

Cuff around bulbar urethra

Control pump in scrotum

Treatment

Conservative

The initial treatment of both UUI and SUI consists of lifestyle advice. Avoiding stimulants (caffeine, fizzy drinks), weight loss, treating constipation and smoking cessation all improve incontinence symptoms. Behavioural therapies such as **timed voiding** (a fixed voiding schedule, for example every 2 hours, which aims to prevent incontinence by providing an opportunity to void before incontinence occurs), **bladder training** (to increase bladder capacity) and **pelvic floor muscle training (PFMT)** have been shown to improve both SUI and UUI. Biofeedback using a perineometer or weighted vaginal cones aid in the teaching of pelvic floor exercises.

Overactive bladder

Pharmacological

Failure of conservative therapies is followed by a trial of pharmacological treatment for OAB. There are two classes of medication that can be used for this condition. **Antimuscarinic agents** (e.g. oxybutynin, solifenacin) are competitive antagonists of the parasympathetic muscarinic acetylcholine receptors on the detrusor muscle, which are normally involved in generating a detrusor contraction. **Beta-3 agonists** (e.g. mirabegron) are agonists of the sympathetic beta-3 adrenergic receptors, thereby allowing detrusor muscle relaxation and reducing OAB symptoms (Figure 10.4).

Surgical

If pharmacological treatments fail to improve symptoms, patients should undergo urodynamic testing prior to more invasive therapies. Second-line options for patients who have failed pharmacological treatment are as follow.
- *Intravesical botulinum toxin A injections:* botulinum toxin A acts on both sensory afferent and motor efferent nerve pathways to reduce the sensation of urgency and to reduce detrusor muscle contractility. It can be injected under local anaesthetic as an outpatient procedure. However, there is a small risk of voiding dysfunction so all patients should be able to perform self-catheterisation in case they are unable to void spontaneously following this treatment. The effect typically lasts 6–12 months and therefore needs repeating if successful (Figure 10.5).
- *Sacral neuromodulation:* this involves the implantation of a 'pacemaker-like' pulse generator which stimulates a tined lead placed predominantly by the S3 nerve root to improve OAB symptoms. Its mechanism of action is not completely understood but approximately 75% of patients with idiopathic detrusor overactivity notice a significant improvement in symptoms (Figure 10.6).
- *Augmentation 'clam' cystoplasty:* a surgical procedure that aims to increase bladder capacity by bivalving the bladder and inserting a segment of detubularised small intestine typically. Patients need to be counselled regarding the risks of surgery, including need for self-catheterisation, recurrent UTI, electrolyte imbalance, stone formation and persistent mucous production.
- *Urinary diversion:* this can be offered as a last resort for patients who have failed or are unsuitable for the other treatment options, and typically involves the creation of an ileal conduit stoma to which the ureters are anastomosed.

Stress incontinence

Female

Currently, the National Institute for Health and Care Excellence (NICE) recommend three main groups of surgical treatments for female SUI that has failed to respond to conservative measures:

1 *Synthetic mid-urethral tape:* the most common procedure for SUI worldwide. It is a minimally invasive procedure with excellent long-term cure rates, which involves the passage of a type I macroporous polypropylene tape under the mid-urethra through an incision in the anterior vaginal wall, thereby reinforcing the sub-urethral vaginal support (Figure 10.7). It can be inserted through the retropubic (tension-free vaginal tape; TVT) or transobturator (TOT) route.

2 *Open colposuspension:* an open surgical procedure that involves approximating the paravaginal fascia either side of the urethra to the ileopectineal (Copper's) ligament using sutures. The aim is to restore the bladder neck to its correct intra-abdominal position allowing any rise in intra-abdominal pressure to be transmitted equally to both the bladder and proximal urethra, resulting in continence.

3 *Autologous fascial sling:* involves harvesting a strip of the patient's own rectus fascia or fascia lata to be used as a sling which is placed at the level of the bladder neck. The advantage is that it avoids the risk of complications that can result from the use of synthetic mesh (such as erosion), but the procedure carries a higher peri-operative morbidity and a higher rate of postoperative voiding dysfunction requiring self-catheterisation.

Other options for the treatment of SUI include:
- *Intraurethral injection of bulking agents:* a procedure with a low operative morbidity but low long-term success rate, generally only offered in selected populations such as the elderly.
- *Artificial urinary sphincter (AUS):* a last resort in female patients who have failed previous surgeries and who have primary urethral sphincter weakness. It involves the placement of a three-piece device, with a cuff around the urethra controlled by a pump that is placed in the labia (women) or scrotum (men) (Figure 10.8). It requires significant patient understanding to operate the device.

Male

SUI in men most commonly occurs as a complication of radical prostatectomy for prostate cancer (post-prostatectomy incontinence). After failure of PFMT, there are two principal surgical treatment options. The **male transobturator sling**, for mild–moderate SUI, causes proximal relocation of the bulb behind the distal sphincter mechanism thereby providing additional support to the existing sphincter. The AUS is used for men with more severe degrees of SUI and is the procedure with the highest long-term success rate and has been around for almost 30 years (Figure 10.8).

Further reading

Abrams P, Cardozo L, Fall M, *et al*; Standardisation Sub-committee of the International Continence Society. The standardisation of terminology of lower urinary tract function: report from the Standardisation Sub-committee of the International Continence Society. *Neurourol Urodyn* 2002; 21: 167–178.

Abrams P, Cardozo L, Khoury S, Wein A. *Incontinence*, 5th edn. International Consultation on Urological Diseases; 2013. http://www.icud.info/incontinence.html (accessed 19 July 2016).

European Association of Urology. *Guidelines on Urinary Incontinence*. www.uroweb.org (accessed 19 July 2016).

11. Neuropathic bladder

Figure 11.1 The neurological control of the lower urinary tract

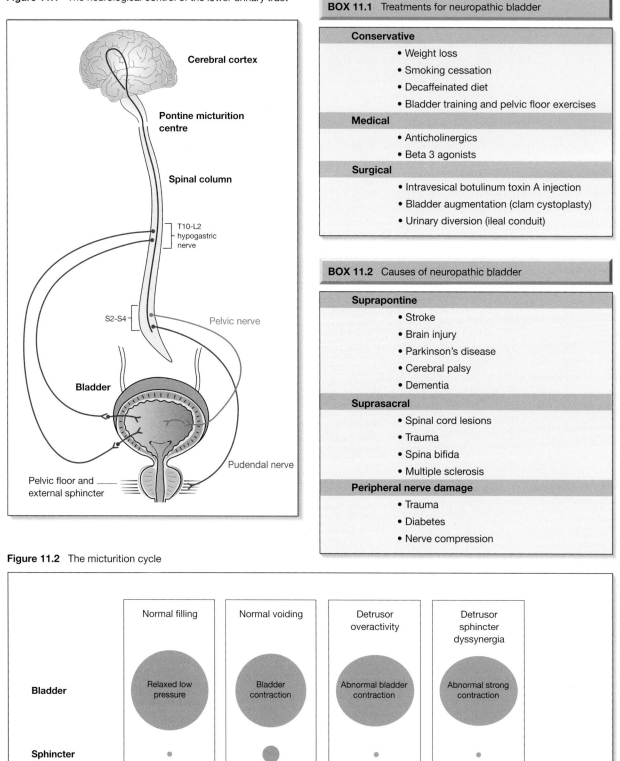

Cerebral cortex

Pontine micturition
centre

Spinal column

T10-L2
hypogastric
nerve

S2-S4

Pelvic nerve

Bladder

Pudendal nerve

Pelvic floor and
external sphincter

BOX 11.1 Treatments for neuropathic bladder

Conservative
- Weight loss
- Smoking cessation
- Decaffeinated diet
- Bladder training and pelvic floor exercises

Medical
- Anticholinergics
- Beta 3 agonists

Surgical
- Intravesical botulinum toxin A injection
- Bladder augmentation (clam cystoplasty)
- Urinary diversion (ileal conduit)

BOX 11.2 Causes of neuropathic bladder

Suprapontine
- Stroke
- Brain injury
- Parkinson's disease
- Cerebral palsy
- Dementia

Suprasacral
- Spinal cord lesions
- Trauma
- Spina bifida
- Multiple sclerosis

Peripheral nerve damage
- Trauma
- Diabetes
- Nerve compression

Figure 11.2 The micturition cycle

	Normal filling	Normal voiding	Detrusor overactivity	Detrusor sphincter dyssynergia
Bladder	Relaxed low pressure	Bladder contraction	Abnormal bladder contraction	Abnormal strong contraction
Sphincter	Closed	Open	Closed	Closed

Urology at a Glance, First Edition. Edited by Hashim Hashim and Prokar Dasgupta. © 2017 John Wiley & Sons, Ltd. Published 2017 by John Wiley & Sons, Ltd.
Companion website: www.ataglanceseries.com/urology

The lower urinary tract has a complex neurological supply involving both the central and peripheral nervous systems. The bladder has both a motor and sensory nerve supply (Figure 11.1).

The micturition cycle

There are two phases:

1 *Filling:* during the filling phase the bladder has to collect sizeable quantities of urine but keep it at low pressure. This is known as bladder compliance and allows bladder filling to occur without the desire to void until the bladder is relatively full.

2 *Voiding:* once it is suitable to void, the gating mechanism inhibiting the detrusor from contracting is overcome and the voiding phase begins. The external urethral sphincter and bladder neck relax and in a coordinated effort the detrusor muscle contacts giving unhindered flow (Figure 11.2).

Neurogenic detrusor overactivity

Neurogenic detrusor overactivity occurs when there is abnormal, unhindered contraction of the detrusor muscle. It can be diagnosed based on symptoms of OAB (urgency with or without incontinence and frequency) and is confirmed by urodynamic testing. The treatment ladder includes lifestyle changes, bladder training, pelvic floor exercises, medications, intravesical botulinum toxin A injection and surgery (Box 11.1).

Lifestyle changes include weight loss and smoking cessation. Dietary modifications include decaffeinated diet and alcohol avoidance as these can increase urination.

Bladder training involves scheduled voiding times with gradually increasing intervals. This helps with control and increases bladder capacity. Over time this normalises the voiding pattern and can help recover the patient's confidence.

Pelvic floor exercises are used to strengthen the pelvic floor and sphincter. This helps with episodes of incontinence and is thought to reduce urgency by inhibiting uncontrolled detrusor contractions.

Anticholinergic medications work by relaxing the detrusor muscle and decreasing its activity. Their side effects include dry mouth, blurred vision, constipation, urinary retention and confusion so patient tolerance can be a problem.

Beta-3 agonists work by stimulating the beta-3 receptor which then relaxes the bladder and increases bladder capacity.

Intravesical botulinum toxin A injections relax the bladder to relieve the symptoms of OAB. They can be performed under general or local anaesthetic but the effect is temporary. There is a risk of urinary retention so patients must be willing and able to perform CISC if this occurs.

Open **surgery** is used in the severest of cases when all other treatments have failed. Bladder augmentation (clam cystoplasty) increases bladder capacity and helps restore bladder normality. Alternatively, a urinary diversion can be performed.

Classification of neuropathic bladder

Suprapontine lesions

Suprapontine lesions affect the neurology of the urinary tract at a level above the pontine micturition centre (PMC). Dementia, cerebrovascular accidents and Parkinson's disease are examples of conditions that can cause this (Box 11.2). Lesions in this area produce functional changes with voiding. They can cause a wide range of symptoms including urge, frequency and detrusor overactivity. Because these lesions are above the PMC, the local micturition sacral reflex arc remains intact leading to normal voiding and a safe low-pressure bladder. However, because there is loss of inhibition from the higher centres of the brain there is neurogenic detrusor overactivity.

Suprasacral lesions

Suprasacral lesions occur between the pons of the brainstem and the L5 spinal segment. Spinal cord injuries, trauma, disc herniation, multiple sclerosis and myelitis can cause these lesions and lead to serious dysfunction of the urinary tract such as detrusor overactivity and sphincter spasticity. This leads to a range of symptoms including urgency, frequency, incomplete bladder emptying (a cause for recurrent urinary tract infections), urinary retention and overflow incontinence. The sphincter spasticity can be so strong that **detrusor sphincter dyssynergia** (DSD) develops. This is when the normal coordinated effect of detrusor contraction and sphincter relaxation is lost. When the bladder is contracting against a closed sphincter, an environment is created where the urinary tract is unsafe leading to high bladder pressures. The bladder then hypertrophies and ureteral reflux occurs. Over time, the function of the kidney can deteriorate.

The mainstay of treatment is to keep bladder pressures low. The simplest way of achieving this, if the patient is capable, is to perform CISC. Sphincterotomy can also be performed but as it is permanent this is usually used as a last resort.

Autonomic dysreflexia is an emergency. In suprasacral lesions above the level of T6, there can be overactvity of the sympathetic nervous system. Provocation by a stimulus below the level of the lesion (e.g. bladder over-distension) leads to pounding headache, abnormal variation in blood pressure (usually hypertension), bradycardia, flushing (above the level of the lesion) and profuse sweating (above the level of the lesion). If this occurs, the patient should be sat up, nifedipine should be given and the stimulus must be removed.

Peripheral nerve lesions S1–S5 (cauda equina)

Lesions at this level lead to loss of tone in the urinary tract. There is an atonic, non-contractile bladder, which has lost its local sacral reflex arc. There is also concurrent loss of sphincter tone leading to stress incontinence. These lesions generally lead to safe, low-pressure bladders.

Further reading

Abrams P. *Urodynamics*, 3rd edn. Springer; 2005.

European Association of Urology (EAU). Neuro-urology. https://uroweb.org/guideline/neuro-urology/ (accessed 20 July 2016).

Hashim H, Abrams P (eds). *Overactive Bladder Syndrome and Urinary Incontinence*. Oxford: Oxford University Press; 2011.

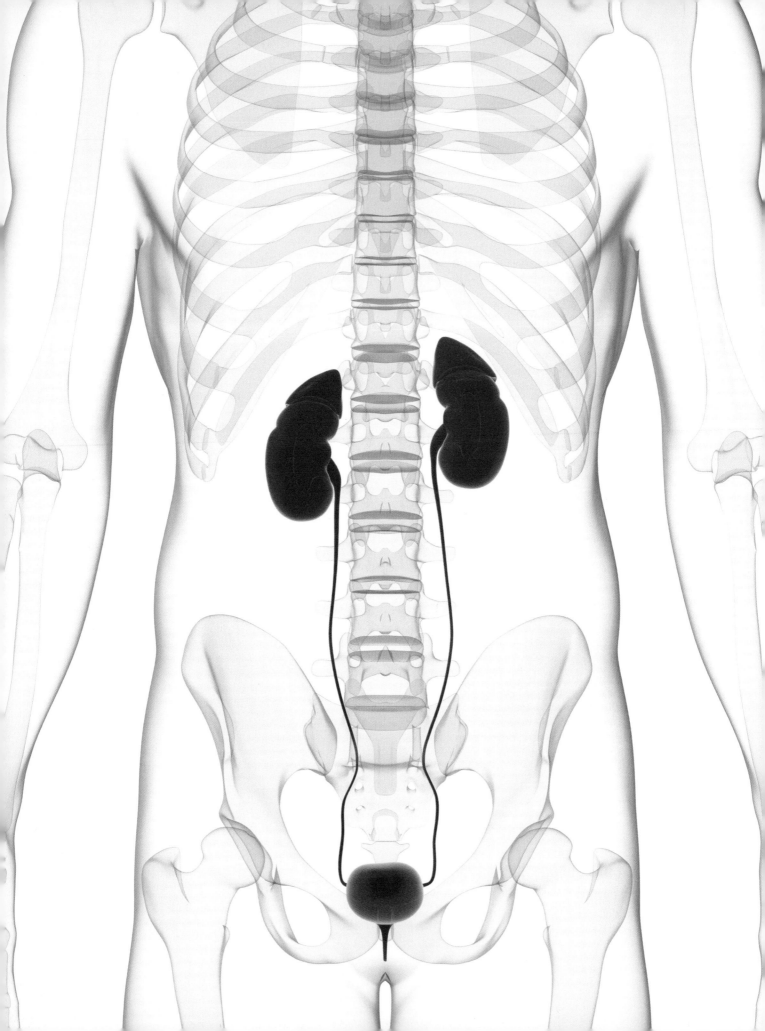

Andrology

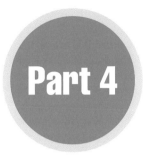

Part 4

Chapters

12 Scrotal swelling and pain

Table 12.1 Classification of scrotal swellings

Emergencies	Malignant	Benign
Torsion	Testicular cancer	Hydrocele
Epididymo-orchitis	Scrotal skin cancer	Epididymal cyst
Trauma	**Benign non-urological**	Sperm granuloma
	Hernia	Varicocele
	Heart failure	Sebaceous cyst

Table 12.2 Scrotal anatomy

Scrotum	Spermatic cord
Scrotal skin	Vas deferens
Dartos muscle	Testicular, scrotal, cremasteric artery
External spermatic fascia	Pampiniform plexus
Cremaster muscle	Lymphatics
Internal spermatic fascia	Genital branch of genitofemoral nerve

Figure 12.1 Scrotal anatomy

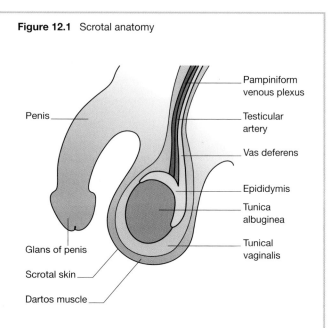

Figure 12.2 Assessing the patient with scrotal pain

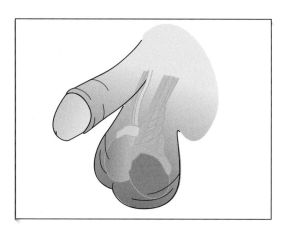

Figure 12.3 Scrotal examination

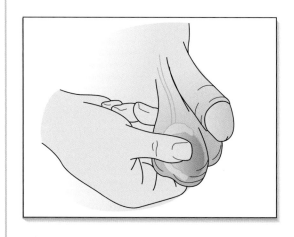

Figure 12.4 Left testicular torsion with ischaemia

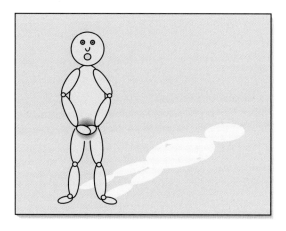

Understanding the causes of a scrotal swelling and scrotal pain

Scrotal pain is either acute, in which case it is deemed a urological emergency, or it can be chronic and intermittent, in which case it can be assessed in an outpatient setting. Patients with acute scrotal pain are often distressed, anxious and need to be assessed immediately to exclude a testicular torsion. This chapter discusses taking the history from the patient, the examination, differential diagnoses for scrotal swellings and scrotal pain and the management for each case. Testicular conditions are categorised into emergencies, malignant and benign causes of testicular swelling (Table 12.1).

Scrotal anatomy See Figure 12.1 and Table 12.2.

Taking the history

Taking the history is the most important step during assessment as it will often lead straight to the underlying diagnosis (Figure 12.2). The patient should be reassured regarding the assessment that will be carried out.

Questions to ask are what type of pain (constant or intermittent) and intensity (1–10 pain scale), location and radiation of pain and, most important, the time of onset (acute or chronic). Ask if any activity triggered the pain and about any associated symptoms such as nausea, vomiting, abdominal or loin pain and urinary frequency.

Query whether there has been any history of recent trauma, unprotected sexual intercourse, history of STIs (particularly gonorrhoea and chlamydia) or systemic infections (mumps orchitis). Remember to ask about any previous surgery or conditions affecting the testes.

Before proceeding to examination, ensure the patient does not have any loin pain or urinary symptoms, as the passage of a ureteric stone (renal colic) can cause pain radiating from the loin to the groin and scrotum (ilioinguinal nerve distribution).

Examination

Examination of the patient should always be carried out with a chaperone present and maintaining the patient's dignity (Figure 12.3). Ensure the patient is in a comfortable, warm environment and has been offered some form of analgesia prior to exposure and examination. The patient's body language will give you a clue about the amount of pain they are in. Reassure them beforehand and explain every step of the examination before starting.

Observation

The patient should lie supine on the examination couch and expose the abdomen, groin and genital area. Observe the position of the testis, swelling or erythema. Compare this with the contralateral side.

Palpation

Examine the non-painful contralateral testis first. Assess position, size and tenderness. When examining the painful testicle, warn the patient first and gently palpate to establish if the testis is tender, and for epididymis and spermatic cord. If there is a scrotal swelling see if you can feel the testis separately and if you can get above the swelling. (You cannot get above the swelling if this is an inguino-scrotal hernia.) At this stage you should try to use a pen torch to see if the swelling transilluminates, suggestive of a hydrocele.

Remember to examine the penis and foreskin too. You can identify a tight foreskin or meatal stricture that can contribute to urinary infections and epididymo-orchitis. Palpate the abdomen and loin areas for localised tenderness and examine the groin

to exclude an inguinal hernia. Always repeat your scrotal examination with the patient standing up and examine the other systems for completeness and review vital signs.

Category A: exclude an emergency
Testicular torsion

This is the most important 'vascular' emergency involving the testis. When the testis is twisted the blood supply is compromised, initially because of venous congestion and then impaired arterial inflow resulting in the development of ischaemia and severe pain (Figure 12.4). The patient often presents with a sudden onset of severe pain in the affected hemiscrotum, sometimes waking them up from sleep. Ask about the time of onset, history of trauma or previous short-lived episodes of a similar pain (indicates an intermittent torsion). The pain often radiates to the groin or even loin because of the nerve distribution (from ilioinguinal nerve, L1 spinal nerve). On examination you may find the testis lies higher than the other one (high-riding) or is lying horizontally because of twisting of the testicle within the tunica vaginalis.

The management for this condition is an immediate scrotal exploration. If the testis is torted then it needs to be untwisted and, if viable, fixed within the scrotum using non-absorbable sutures. This procedure is called orchidopexy and the contralateral testis will have to be fixed as well during the same operation as the risk of testicular torsion on the contralateral side is approximately 30%. Remember that once ischaemia sets in, the testis is viable for only up to 6 hours.

Torsion of a testicular appendage (or hydatid of Morgagni) can sometimes occur with a similar history. A twisted hydatid of Morgagni (vestigial remnant of Müllerian duct) lies on the upper pole of the testis and can sometimes be seen as a 'blue dot' under the scrotal skin in young patients. This also requires surgical exploration and can easily be excised from the testis with diathermy.

Testicular trauma

Testicular trauma occurs with direct or indirect injury, either in sports or from bicycle and road traffic accidents. A scrotal haematoma may be present and the assessment of the genital area remains the same, with the addition of exclusion of pelvic and urethral injuries. In cases where testicular rupture (rupture of the tunica albuginea with extrusion of testicular contents) is suspected, senior review is needed immediately. Ultrasound examination can usually assess whether the tunica albuginea is intact. Scrotal exploration and closure of the tunica albuginea may be required.

Infection of the testis or epididymis

Orchitis (infection of the testis) or epididymo-orchitis (infection of the testis and epididymis) are a common presentation in urology clinics. Patients with infection usually present with scrotal pain, swelling, erythema of the skin and urinary frequency and dysuria, with or without penile discharge. In patients over 50 years exclude the presence of bladder outlet obstruction triggering a UTI. In younger patients exclude an STI. These patients usually present with epididymitis (inflammation and bulkiness of the epididymis only). If there are signs of sepsis admit the patient to a ward and start intravenous antibiotics. Antibiotic treatment, both oral and intravenous, should be instigated according to the hospital's guidelines.

Fournier's gangrene is a real emergency but rarely seen. It is a necrotising fasciitis of the external genitalia skin, occurring in patients with scrotal skin infection or UTI. Predisposing factors are diabetes and diseases affecting the immune system. This condition requires immediate resuscitation, senior review, surgical debridement and escalation to a high-dependency unit postoperatively.

Figure 12.5 Testicular tumour

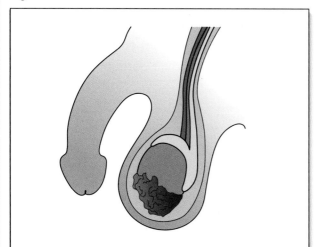

Table 12.3 Testicular cancer

Germ cell tumours (GCT) (90%)	Other tumours (7%)
Seminoma (48%)	Lymphoma (5%)
Non-seminomatous GCT (INSCT) (42%)	Rare
• Embryonal carcinoma • Yolk sac tumour • Choriocarcinoma • Teratoma • Mixed GCT	• Adenomatoid tumour • Adenocarcinoma of the rete rete testis • Carcinoid • Metastatic from other side
Mixed GCT (10%)	
Sex cord stromal tumours (3%)	Leydig, Sertoli cell tumours, mixed

Figure 12.6 Hydrocele

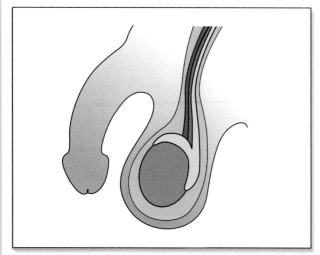

Figure 12.7 Epididymal cyst

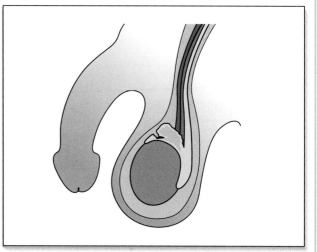

Figure 12.8 Sperm granuloma post vasectomy

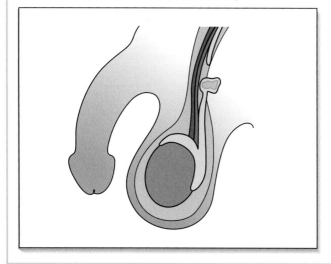

Figure 12.9 Varicocele

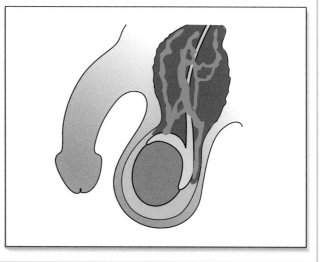

Category B: malignant causes of scrotal swelling

Testicular tumour

Most patients with testicular tumour present with a painless scrotal lump. Testicular swelling can occur rapidly over a few days or weeks, sometimes with an associated hydrocele. Only 20% of patients present with testicular pain which can be acute if there has been a bleed from the tumour. Taking a complete history is important, particularly asking about a history of undescended testes or a family history. The lump can feel irregular and hard and will arise from the testicle itself. A general examination should be followed by an ultrasound scan of the scrotum which is very accurate in diagnosing testicular tumours (Figure 12.5; Table 12.3).

Management includes serum tumour markers (alpha fetoprotein, human chorionic gonadotrophin, lactic dehydrogenase), discussion in the multi-disciplinary team meeting and urgent inguinal radical orchidectomy after sperm banking. A staging CT of the chest–abdomen–pelvis should be carried out to exclude metastatic disease as testicular tumours metastasise to the para-aortic lymph nodes but cure rates are >95%.

Category C: benign causes of scrotal swelling

Most patients presenting to the urology clinic with scrotal swellings are found to have benign conditions.

Hydrocele

A hydrocele is an abnormal collection of fluid contained within the tunica vaginalis (remnant piece of peritoneum around the testis; Figure 12.6). It is difficult or even impossible to palpate the testis within the swelling but if you can get above the swelling and it transilluminates then this is diagnostic of a hydrocele.

Hydroceles are easily diagnosed using ultrasound which can occasionally pick up an underlying testicular tumour if the hydrocele has occurred over a short period of time.

If the testis is normal and the patient is symptomatic because of a large hydrocele then a surgical repair can be offered. Aspiration techniques have been abandoned because of the high recurrence rate, but can be appropriate for patients unsuitable for surgery. Most patients undergo a procedure whereby the hydrocele is drained with an incision followed by eversion (Jaboulay's procedure) or plication (Lord's procedure) of the tunica vaginalis to prevent recurrence.

Epididymal cyst

Epididymal cysts are cystic swellings found on the epididymal head and some contain fluid or even spermatozoa (Figure 12.7). If they contain spermatozoa they are called **spermatoceles**. Patients can present at any age. When cysts are large they can cause pain or a dragging sensation in the scrotum. The lump is felt separate from the testis but is part of the epididymis. When cysts are large they can also transilluminate.

If symptomatic, a surgical excision can be offered to the patient but, as with any operation, there are risks, such as postoperative haematoma or infection, recurrence of the cyst and, rarely, scarring of the epididymis causing impaired fertility or chronic pain (fewer than 1 in 50).

Sperm granuloma

A sperm granuloma is benign and occurs mainly after a vasectomy at the cut ends of the vas deferens (Figure 12.8). Excision is only performed if this is large or symptomatic when patients complain of ongoing post-vasectomy pain.

Varicocele

A varicocele is a dilatation of the veins of the pampiniform plexus in the spermatic cord, most commonly on the left-hand side because the left spermatic vein enters the renal vein at a right angle resulting in higher pressures (Figure 12.9). The right vein enters the inferior vena cava directly.

The dilatation occurs as a result of incompetent valves in the internal spermatic veins. Most patients are asymptomatic but large varicoceles can cause pain or a heavy feeling in the scrotum. When examined varicoceles feel like a 'bag of worms' and become more prominent when the patient stands up or on Valsalva manoeuvre. These patients need to be assessed for infertility as this occurs in about 25% of patients. Any acute varicocele presentation should be followed by a renal ultrasound scan to exclude a tumour causing extrinsic pressure on the venous system.

If intervention is required, surgical ligation of the veins or embolisation by interventional radiology can be offered.

Benign non-urological causes of scrotal swelling

Inguino-scrotal hernia

An indirect inguinal hernia often extends into the scrotum and so is called an inguino-scrotal hernia. This presents as a scrotal swelling where the doctor cannot get above the swelling on examination which differentiates it from a hydrocele. This condition in managed by the General Surgeons and when pain occurs, strangulation of the hernia needs to be excluded.

Heart failure

Patients with heart failure have fluid retention with oedema and swelling of the legs. Occasionally, you will encounter patients with bilateral symmetrical scrotal swelling as well. The scrotal skin is oedematous and sometimes there is also erythema. It is difficult to establish this diagnosis in some patients and a general examination with ultrasound assessment of the scrotum is required. The ultrasound will report soft tissue swelling and can exclude a hydrocele and assess the testis too. These patients do not need follow-up by a urologist but should be referred to the cardiology department. The scrotal swelling usually settles with improvement of heart failure.

Ultrasound of the scrotum

Ultrasound of the scrotum is the best radiological technique to provide a final diagnosis of a testicular swelling and cause of pain. It can be carried out quickly and in expert hands it is diagnostic for all the pathologies mentioned in this chapter except testicular torsion.

Testicular torsion is a clinical diagnosis. A Doppler ultrasound can review the blood supply in the testis if there is suspicion that a torsion occurred more than 12 hours ago and the testis is not viable. In the acute setting an ultrasound scan is not indicated and should not delay surgical exploration.

Further reading

European Association of Urology (EAU). Guidelines on Testicular Cancer. 2015. http://uroweb.org/wp-content/uploads/EAU-Guidelines-Testicular-Cancer-2015-v2.pdf (accessed 20 July 2016).

Reynard J, Brewster S, Biers S. *Oxford Handbook of Urology*, 3rd edn. Oxford: Oxford University Press; 2013.

World Health Organization (WHO). Histological Classification of Testis Tumours. http://www.iarc.fr/en/publications/pdfs-online/pat-gen/bb7/bb7-chap4.pdf (accessed 20 July 2016).

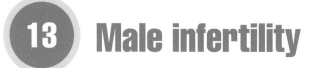

13 Male infertility

Table 13.1 Evaluation of the infertile male

Infertility history	Medical
Duration • Prior conceptions • Current or previous partner • Outcome Previous fertility evaluation and treatment	Diabetes mellitus Neurological disease • Spinal cord injury • Multiple sclerosis Infection • Urinary infections • Sexually transmitted disease • Epididymitis/prostatitis • Tuberculosis • Mumps orchitis • Recent viral/febrile illness Renal disease Cancer • Chemotherapy/radiotherapy
Sexual history	
Erectile function Lubricants Frequency/timing of intercourse	
Past history	**Surgical**

Childhood
• Cryptorchidism
• Onset of puberty
• Testicular pathology
  ○ Torsion
  ○ Trauma
• Midline defects (cleft palate)
	Orchidopexy
	Retroperitoneal/pelvic surgery
	Herniorrhaphy
	Vasectomy
	Bladder neck/prostatic surgery

Family history	**Medications**
Infertility Cystic fibrosis Androgen receptor deficiency	Gonadotoxins • Environmental exposures (pesticides, heavy metals) • Radiation • Habits (tobacco, recreational drugs, anabolic steroids)

Table 13.2 Lower reference limits (5th centiles and their 95% confidence intervals) for semen. Characteristics *adapted from WHO reference values for semen analysis*

Parameter	Lower reference limit (range)
Semen volume (mL)	1.5 (1.4–1.7)
Total sperm number (10^6 per mL)	39 (33–46)
Sperm concentration (10^6 per ejaculate)	15 (12–16)
Total motility (PR + NP)	40 (38–42)
Progressive motility (PR, %)	32 (31–34)
Vitality (live spermatozoa, %)	58 (55–63)
Sperm morphology (normal forms, %)	4 (3.0–4.0)
Other consensus threshold values	
pH > 7.2	
Peroxidase-positive leucocytes (106 per mL)	<1.0
MAR test (motile spermatozoa with bound particles, %)	<50
Immunobead test (motile spermatozoa with bound beads, %)	<50
Seminal zinc (mol/ejaculate)	>2.4
Seminal fructose (mol/ejaculate)	>13
Seminal neutral glucosidase (mU/ejaculate)	>20
Semen volume (mL)	1.5 (1.4–1.7)

MAR, mixed antiglobulin reaction; NP, non-progressive; PR, progressive.

Figure 13.1 The hypothalamic-pituitry-gonadal axis

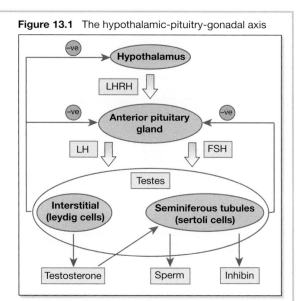

Box 13.1 Aetiology

Pre-testicular causes:

1 Endocrinopathy/hormonal, hypogonadotropic hypogonadism
2 Systemic disease (e.g. renal failure; liver cirrhosis; cystic fibrosis)
3 Environmental factors (e.g. hot baths)
4 Drugs, alcohol and smoking
5 Genetic abnormalities.

Testicular causes:

1 Varicocele present in 40%
2 Idiopathic 25%
3 Undescended testes (cryptorchidism)
4 Functional sperm disorder (e.g. antisperm antibodies, Kartagener's syndrome)
5 Testicular injury (e.g. testicular torsion)
6 Infection (e.g. post-pubertal mumps orchitis)
7 Radiation
8 Cancer
9 Genetic disorder (e.g. Kleinfelter's syndrome).

Post-testicular (obstructive causes):

1 Male genital tract obstruction (e.g. obstruction/absence of vas deferens)
2 Erectile or ejaculatory problems (e.g. retrograde ejaculation)
3 Infection (e.g. prostatitis).

Urology at a Glance, First Edition. Edited by Hashim Hashim and Prokar Dasgupta. © 2017 John Wiley & Sons, Ltd. Published 2017 by John Wiley & Sons, Ltd.
Companion website: www.ataglanceseries.com/urology

Male infertility refers to a male's inability to achieve pregnancy. The introduction of intra-cytoplasmic sperm injection (ICSI) in 1992 was a revolution in the management of male infertility.

Definitions

1 Subfertility: failure of conception after at least 12 months of regular unprotected intercourse.

2 Azoospermia: the absence of sperm in the ejaculate which is identified in 10–15% of infertile males.

3 Oligospermia: a sperm density of <20 million/mL. Unlike the situation with azoospermia, causes of oligospermia can be vast and the aetiology is often idiopathic.

4 Asthenospermia: decreased sperm mobility (<32% motile spermatozoa).

5 Teratospermia: abnormal forms of sperm (<4% normal forms).

Sperm abnormalities of 3, 4 and 5 usually occur together and are termed oligo-astheno-teratozoospermia (OAT) syndrome.

In 50% of infertile couples, a male infertility associated factor is found together with abnormal semen parameters.

Physiology

The hypothalamic–pituitary–gonadal (HPG) axis is responsible for reproductive tract formation and development, maturation of fertility potential at puberty and the maintenance of maleness in the adult (Figure 13.1).

Aetiology

The male factor contributes to infertility in approximately 50% of cases. The most common causes are a problem in the production or delivery of sperm. Up to 25% of cases are idiopathic (i.e. no cause will be found); however, in other cases the causes are reversible, see Box 13.1.

History

A through history taking is the key in successful diagnosis of male infertility (Table 13.1).

Examination

General examination

Perform a comprehensive general examination with particular attention to: evidence of secondary sexual development; gynaecomastia; signs of hypogonadism; decreased body hair, absence of temporal pattern balding areas; disproportionately long extremities due to delayed closure of the epiphyseal plates caused by low androgen levels at the time of puberty; examination of thyroid gland to rule out nodules suggesting hyperfunction or hypofunction, which can affect fertility; hepatomegaly on abdominal examination raises suspicion for hepatic dysfunction, which can induce altered sex steroid metabolism.

Genital examination

- *Penis:* curvature, Peyronie's plaque, phimosis, hypospadias
- *Testes:* measurement of testicular consistency, tenderness and volume (using orchidometer or sonographic measurement; normally >20 mL)
- *Epididymis:* tenderness and swelling
- *Spermatic cord:* presence or absence of vas deferens, varicocele
- *Digital rectal examination of prostate:* Müllerian duct cysts, tenderness, palpable seminal vesicles.

Investigations

Basic investigations

Appropriate laboratory testing of semen has a key role in evaluation of men presenting with infertility.

1 *Semen analysis:* 2–3 specimens should be collected over the period of few weeks after 3–7 days of sexual abstinence. The specimen should be delivered to the laboratory within 1 hour. Normal parameters of semen analysis are shown in Table 13.2.

2 *Hormonal assessment:* these include luteinising hormone (LH), follicle stimulating hormone (FSH) and testosterone. Increased prolactin level is associated with sexual dysfunction and can indicate pituitary disease.

Special investigations

1 Genetic studies including karyotype analysis, Y chromosome microdeletion and cystic fibrosis transmembrane conductance regulator status.

2 In selected cases, testicular biopsy can be indicated to exclude spermatogenic failure (non-obstructive causes).

3 Post-orgasmic urine analysis.

4 Sperm function tests (rarely used): post coital test; sperm penetration test; sperm–cervical mucus test.

Radiological investigations

1. Ultrasound scan of the scrotum to assess testicular volume, abnormality and the presence of varicoceles.

2. Transrectal ultrasound of prostate and seminal vesicles if sperm volume is low to rule out obstructive causes.

3. Vasography: a contrast study where contrast is injected into the vas deferens through a puncture in the scrotum. This is to diagnose and evaluate the level of obstruction.

4. Venography for the diagnosis and treatment (embolisation) of varicocele.

Management

Treatments vary according to the underlying cause and the degree of impairment. Pre-testicular conditions and idiopathic cases may respond to medical therapy:

- **Gonadotropin-releasing hormone agonists:** these agents are effective for treatment of hypogonadotropic hypogonadism.
- **Anti-oestrogens** remain the most commonly employed medical therapy for idiopathic male infertility (e.g. clomiphene citrate and tamoxifen citrate).
- **Antioxidant therapy:** vitamins E and C.

Testicular conditions (and idiopathic infertility that does not respond to medical treatment) could be treated with assisted reproduction techniques (ART).

Sperm extraction from the epididymis is performed by: percutanenous epididymal sperm aspiration (PESA); microsurgical epididymal sperm aspiration (MESA); testicular exploration and sperm extraction (TESE) or aspiration (TESA).

The retrieved sperm is stored by cryopreservation until required for assisted conception by the following procedures: intrauterine insemination (IUI); *in vitro* fertilisation (IVF); gamete intra-fallopian transfer (GIFT); ICSI.

Post-testicular conditions can be managed with either surgery or IVF-ICSI. Epididymal obstruction can be treated by vasoepididymostomy. Vas deferens obstruction can be overcome by vasovasostomy. Ejaculatory duct obstruction requires transurethral resection of the ejaculatory ducts (TURED).

Varicoceles are treated by embolisation, open, laparoscopic or microsurgical operations. Erectile dysfunction is treated conventionally by medications, vacuum devices or prosthesis. Ejaculatory conditions can be treated by medication, or by IUI therapy or IVF.

Further reading

Jarow JP, Espeland MA, Lipshultz LI. Evaluation of the azoospermic patient. *J Urol* 1989; 142: 62–65.

Jungwirth A, Giwercman A, Tournaye H, *et al.* European Association of Urology guidelines on male infertility: The 2012 update. *Eur Urol* 2012; 62: 324–332.

Palermo G, Joris H, Devroey P, Van Steirteghem AC. Pregnancies after intracytoplasmic injection of single spermatozoon into an oocyte. *Lancet* 1992; 340: 17–18.

14 Erectile dysfunction

Table 14.1 Causes of erectile dysfunction

Physical causes:

Vasculogenic: Hypertension, hyperlipidaemia, diabetes mellitus, peripheral vascular disease, smoking, impairment of cavernosal veno-occlusive mechanism, mixed

Neurogenic: Multiple sclerosis, Parkinsons disease, spina bifida, spinal cord injury, tumour, pelvic surgery or radiotherapy, peripheral neuropathy (diabetes, alcohol-related)

Endocrinological: Hypogonadism, hyperprolactinaemia, hypo- or hyperparathyroidism, diabetes mellitus

Medications: Antihypertensives (β-blockers, thiazides, ACE inhibitors), anti-arrythmics (aminodarone), antidepressants, (tricyclics, MAOIs, SSRIs), anxiolytics (benzodiazepine), anti-androgens (finasteride, cyproterone acetate), GnRH analogues, anticonvulsants, (phenytoin, carbamazepine), anti-Parkinson drugs (levodopa), statins

Mechanical: Peyronie's disease

Trauma: Pelvic fracture, spinal cord injury, penile fracture/trauma

Inflammatory: Prostatitis

Latrogenic: Pelvic surgery, prostatectomy

Psychological causes

Generalised: Generalised unresponsiveness, primary lack of sexual arousability, aging-related decline in sexual arousability

Situational: Lack of arousability in specific relationship, performance related, depression

Nerve supply

• *Central*: higher centres for penile erection and sexual functions are located in the hypothalamus. The medial pre-optic area and paraventricular nucleus in the hypothalamus are considered significant centres.

• *Somatic*: the dorsal penile and pudendal nerves carry the afferent fibres to the spinal cord at S2–S4 level. Efferent information travels from Onuf 's nucleus (S2–S4) to penile ischiocavernosus and bulbocavernosus muscles.

• *Autonomic*: parasympathetic stimulation is responsible for erection whereas sympathetic causes ejaculation. The parasympathetic fibres originating from sacral segments S2–S4 and the sympathetic from the level of T11–L2 join to form the pelvic plexus and then the cavernosal nerves (parasympathetic fibres) originate from pelvic plexus and innervate the penis.

Figure 14.1 Nerve supply and cellular physiology

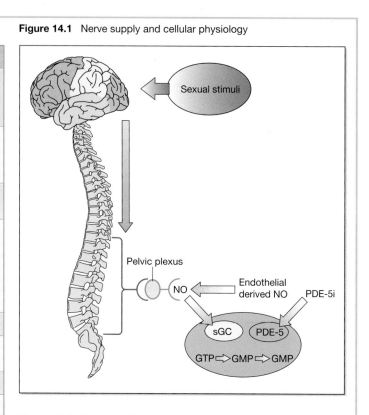

Figure 14.2 Cross-sectional anatomy of penis

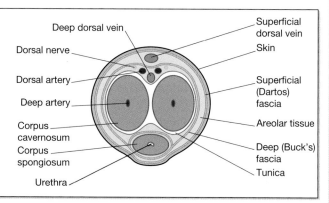

Figure 14.3 Penile anatomy

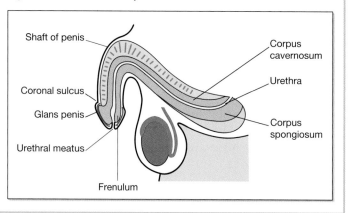

Urology at a Glance, First Edition. Edited by Hashim Hashim and Prokar Dasgupta. © 2017 John Wiley & Sons, Ltd. Published 2017 by John Wiley & Sons, Ltd.
Companion website: www.ataglanceseries.com/urology

Erectile dysfunction (ED), also known as impotence, is the consistent or recurrent inability to attain or maintain a penile erection sufficiently for satisfactory sexual intercourse. It ranges from partial decrease in penile rigidity to a complete erectile failure.

Physiology of penile erection

(Figures 14.1, 14.2 and 14.3)

Haemodynamics of penile erection

The paired internal pudendal artery is the major carrier of the blood supply to the penis. This artery is terminally divided into three branches: the bulbo-urethral, dorsal and cavernous arteries. The cavernous artery supplies the corpora cavernosa; the dorsal artery, the skin, subcutaneous tissue and the glans penis; and the bulbo-urethral artery, the corpus spongiosum.

Activation of the autonomic nerve produces a full erection, that is filling and trapping of blood in the cavernous bodies. After full erection is achieved, contraction of the ischiocavernosus muscle (from activation of the somatic nerves) compresses the proximal corpora and raises the pressure in the entire corpora well above the systolic blood pressure, resulting in rigid erection.

Anatomic mechanism of penile erection

During erection, dilatation of the arterial tree, expansion of the sinusoids and the compression of the subtunical and emissary veins occur. The intrinsic smooth muscle tone and possibly the adrenergic tonic discharge maintain contraction of the smooth muscles and the arterioles in the flaccid state. When the smooth muscles relax owing to release of neurotransmitters, the resistance to incoming flow drops to a minimum. This allows arterial and arteriolar vasodilatation and expansion of the sinusoids to receive a large increase of flow. Trapping of blood causes the penis to lengthen and widen rapidly until the capacity of the tunica albuginea is reached. Meanwhile, expansion of the sinusoidal walls against one another and against the tunica albuginea results in compression of the subtunical venular plexus. Uneven stretching of the layers of the tunica albuginea also compresses the emissary veins and effectively reduces the venous flow to a minimum.

Causes of male erectile dysfunction

The causes of ED are multifactorial (Box 14.1). Organic factors such as chronic medical conditions including hypertension, diabetes mellitus, as well as adverse effects of therapies used for these conditions are known to constitute major causes of ED.

Evidence suggests that there is a strong association between age and ED. This is because cardiovascular risk factors are associated with increasing age and, since penile erection is primarily a vascular event, it can be impaired in conditions in which degenerative changes result in endothelial dysfunction.

Furthermore, the physiological alterations related to hormonal changes and sedentary lifestyle have been implicated in the causes of ED. It is also reported that psychological problems such as depression, performance anxiety and relationship problems could be both complications and risk factors for ED. Inappropriately treated priapism can lead to ED, particularly the ischaemic type.

Treatment

Various risk factors can lead to ED, some of which are reversible. Lifestyle changes are important in individuals with ED, particularly in diabetes and hypertension. They can also improve overall cardiovascular and metabolic conditions. Most of the causes can be treated successfully with current treatment options but cannot be cured except for psychogenic and hormonal causes (e.g. hypogonadism and hyperprolactinaemia). Psychosexual therapy sessions are arranged for patients with non-organic ED. Replacement therapy for testosterone may be effective in testicular failure. DRE, PSA, haematocrit, liver function tests and lipid profile should be checked before starting testosterone replacement therapy. ED secondary to hormonal causes can be cured with specific treatments.

Once conservative treatment fails, the next line of therapy is oral medication. Three potent selective phosphodiesterase E-5 inhibitors (PDE-5i) are available. They are not initiators of erection and require sexual stimulation for an erection to occur. The choice of a PDE-5i depends on the frequency of intercourse and the patient's personal experience.

Sildenafil (Viagra) is effective following 30–60 min administration; a heavy, fatty meal can reduce or prolong absorption. Tadalafil (Cialis) is effective after 30 min after aministration but its peak efficacy occurs after about 2 hours. Efficacy is maintained for up to 36 hours and is not affected by food. It is also considered to be more effective in diabetic patients. Vardenafil (Levitra) is effective 30 min after administration. Vacuum erection devices (VED) can be useful; they apply a negative pressure to draw venous blood into the penis. VED need a motivated patient and an understanding partner as most patients discontinue use within 3 months.

Common side effects of PDE-5i include headache, flushing, dizziness, dyspepsia and nasal congestion.

Sildenafil and vardenafil have been associated with visual abnormalities, while tadalafil has been associated with back pain and myalgia. Due to unpredictable hypotension, nitrates are contraindicated with PDE-5i. Similarly, alpha-blockers interact and can result in orthostatic hypotension.

If oral therapy fails, the next line of treatment is intracavernous injections. Alprostadil is associated with success rates of up to 85%. One or two visits are required to learn the technique by the patient or even by the partner. Complications include penile pain, prolonged erections, priapism and fibrosis.

Some patients prefer intra-urethral alprostadil (MUSE) as a semi-solid pellet. A vascular interaction between the urethra and the corpora cavernosa enables drug transfer between these structures Side effects include local pain, dizziness and urethral bleeding. There is now a cream form of alprostadil which is applied to the tip of the penis.

Priapism occurs very rarely after treatment for ED (<1%). However, most men with ED secondary to priapism do not respond to oral medications and are best treated surgically with a penile prosthesis. Surgical implantation of a penile prosthesis can be considered in patients who fail pharmacotherapy or who want a permanent solution. Complications include mechanical failures and infections.

Further reading

British Society for Sexual Medicine (BSSM). Guidelines on the management of erectile dysfunction. http://www.bssm.org.uk/downloads/BSSM_ED_Management_Guidelines_2013.pdf (accessed 20 July 2016).

European Association of Urology (EAU). Guidelines on male sexual dysfunction. http://uroweb.org/wp-content/uploads/14-Male-Sexual-Dysfunction_LR1.pdf (accessed 20 July 2016).

Muneer A, Kalsi J, Nazareth I, Arya M. Erectile dysfunction. *BMJ* 2014; 348: g129.

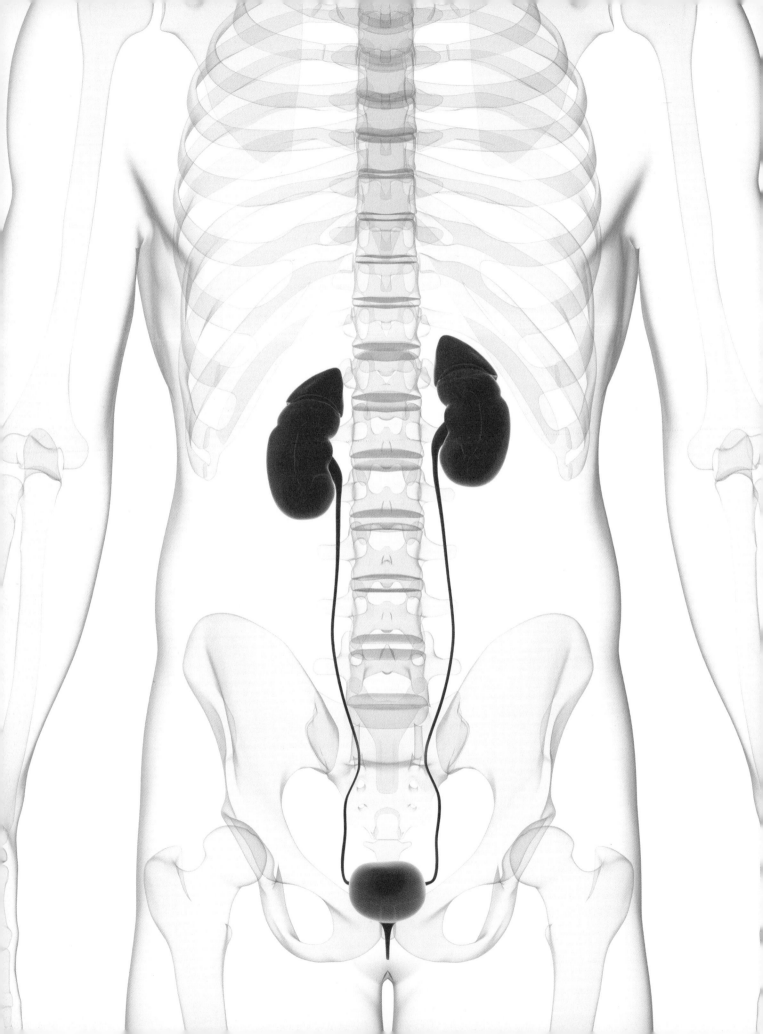

Urological cancers

Part 5

Chapters

15 Urological malignancies

Figure 15.1 Average number of new cases per year and age-specific incidence rates per 100,000 population, males,UK.
Source: Cancer Research UK, http://www.cancerresearchuk.org/sites/default/files/cstream-node/cases_crude_prostate_1.pdf. Accessed June 2016

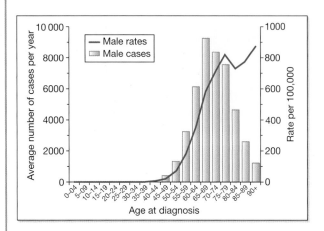

Figure 15.2 The original Gleason grading system was 1–5 giving scores of 2–10, but this has now been reclassified and we only use Gleason 3–5 givingscores of 6–10. Source Epstein 2016; 40: 244-252. Reproduced with permission of *The American Journal of Surgical Pathology* and Lippincott Williams & Wilkins

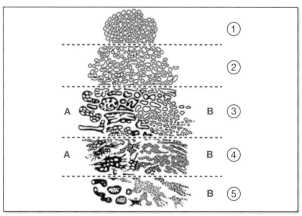

Figure 15.3 MRI of prostate gland with arrow indicating area which was proven to be Gleason 7 Carcinoma of prostate

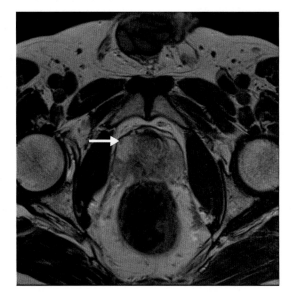

Figure 15.4 Transrectal ultrasound of the prostate prior to biopsy for elevated PSA: longitudinal and sagittal views

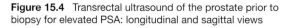
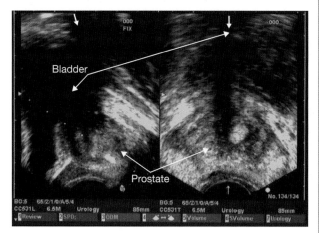

Table 15.1 Age-specific PSA

Age range	PSA cut off (ng/mL)
40–49	<2.5
50–59	<3.5
60–69	<4.5
70–79	<6.5

Table 15.2 TNM staging for prostate cancer

T1	Tumour is too small to be seen or felt
T2	Tumour is within the prostate gland and has not breached the capsule
T3	Tumour has breached the prostate capsule and may have invaded the seminal vesicles
T4	Tumour has invaded other organs

N0	No lymph node involvement
N1	Lymph node involvement
M0	No metastases
M1	Metastases

Urology at a Glance, First Edition. Edited by Hashim Hashim and Prokar Masgupta. © 2017 John Wiley & Sons, Ltd. Published 2017 by John Wiley & Sons, Ltd.
Companion website: www.ataglanceseries.com/urology

Prostate cancer

Prostate cancer is the most common cancer in men in the UK with an incidence of approximately 130 per 100,000 men which equates to a lifetime risk of 1 in 8.

Risk factors

- *Age:* increasing incidence with age
- *Ethnicity:* higher rate in black men
- *Family history:* first degree relatives, carriage of the *BRCA* gene associated with breast cancer in women.

Prostate cancer presentation has been revolutionised by the tumour marker PSA and although the UK government does not currently advocate screening for prostate cancer (based on the outcome of two large multi-centre studies), an increasing number of men are diagnosed through PSA testing while asymptomatic.

PSA is not a perfect test for screening. It can be elevated in:
- Benign prostatic enlargement (BPE)
- Infection
- Trauma (e.g. catheterisation or biopsy).

Most centres now use age-specific PSA to assess patients as PSA rises with age (Figure 15.1).

Prostate cancer can also be diagnosed by rectal examination.

Investigations

Once a man has been found to have an elevated PSA the next step is a prostate biopsy. This can be performed either transrectally or transperineally and allows tissue to be obtained to make a histological diagnosis. Some centres now perform an MRI scan of the prostate prior to biopsy to provide better targeting for biopsies.

Histologically, prostate cancer is an adenocarcinoma derived from the epithelial cells of the prostate, but very rarely primary small cell tumours or metastases.

Adenocarcinoma of the prostate is assigned a Gleason score depending on how the cellular architecture appears under the microscope (Figure 15.2).

Patients can also present with the symptoms of more advanced prostate cancer, typically bone pain or haematuria with or without symptoms of BOO.

For men who present with a grossly elevated PSA and who are elderly, sometimes a bone scan only is performed for diagnosis to prevent the need for a prostate biopsy with its attendant risks of infection.

Once a histological or clinical diagnosis of prostate cancer is made, staging investigations are performed. These usually take the form of
- Bone scan
- MRI scan of the pelvis.

Planning treatment for men with prostate cancer depends upon their Gleason score and staging (Figures 15.3 and 15.4).

The TNM classification is used (Tables 15.1 and 15.2). Using this classification, men with prostate cancer are broadly divided into three groups:
1 Localised: the tumour is within the prostate and has not spread
2 Locally advanced (T3): the tumour has spread locally but is not metastatic
3 Metastatic.

Treatment

In **localised prostate cancer,** patients are often offered a choice of treatment depending on their age, health and the Gleason score of the tumour:
- *Active surveillance:* the tumour is monitored with regular PSA, rectal exam, biopsy and MRI. This is only suitable for men who have tumours that do not appear to be too aggressive. Not all patients are suitable for active surveillance; they need to have a PSA <10, Gleason score <7 and <25% of their biopsy involved with cancer. Some centres also use the amount of cancer visible on MRI to help determine suitability.
- *Radical prostatectomy:* removal of the whole of the prostate gland. This can be performed open, laparoscopically or robotically. It carries a risk of impotence and urinary incontinence. Patients undergoing this are usually expected to have at least a 10-year life expectancy.
- *Radical radiotherapy:* external beam radiation treatment carries a risk of impotence, radiation proctitis and incontinence as a result of radiation cystitis or sphincter rigidity. It is quite often coupled with hormonal manipulation for between 6 months and 3 years depending upon the patient's risk factors.
- *Brachytherapy:* implantation of radioactive seeds. Carries similar risks to external beam radiation.
- *High intensity focused ultrasound:* uses ultrasound to destroy part of the prostate, not widely available. Can reduce the side effect risk, but may not be as effective oncologically.
- *Cryotherapy:* uses freezing to kill the prostate cancer cells. Carries similar risks to external beam radiation and can lead to fistula formation, but only small numbers are performed.
- *Watchful waiting:* generally reserved for men who are very elderly or unfit and therefore likely to die from another disease process. This means not instituting treatment at the time of diagnosis, but waiting for the patient to develop symptoms from the disease or its metastases and then instituting hormonal manipulation with the aim of keeping the disease under control (see Metastatic disease).

In **locally advanced disease,** most patients are offered **radical radiotherapy** although some choose to undergo **radical surgery** or **watchful waiting.**

Metastatic disease by definition is incurable, and patients undergo a variety of treatments to palliate their symptoms, the mainstay of which is hormonal manipulation. In recent years newer treatments like chemotherapy (docetaxel) and forms of hormone manipulation (abiraterone, enzalutamide) have become available once first-line hormone treatment fails.

Hormone manipulation

Prostate cancer grows on the male sex hormone testosterone, hormone manipulation reduces the testosterone level either by blocking it locally at the cellular level (bicalutamide, cyproterone) or by causing the pituitary–hypothalamic axis to be switched off so no testosterone is produced from the testes (LHRH agonists and antagonists). Most patients respond to this treatment well and some can live a number of years with their metastatic disease.

Not all prostate cancers require treatment and it can be a difficult task for the clinician and patient to select who will benefit.

Figure 15.5 (a) The Bosniak classification of cystic renal masses L, liver; K, kidney

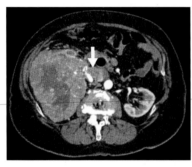

I: 'Simple' (uncomplicated) cyst: smooth, well-defined wall, round/oval, no internal echoes, posterior acoustic shadow → Benign

II: Minimally complicated: <3 cm, septa, calcification, hyperdense (may contain blood) → 5% malignant

IIF: >3 cm or more septa: follow-up imaging required

III: Complicated: irregular margin, thickened septa, thick irregular calcification → 50% malignant

IV: Large, irregular cystic margins with solid internal components → >90% malignant

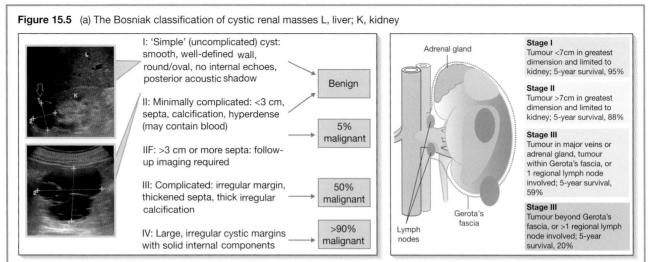

Stage I
Tumour <7cm in greatest dimension and limited to kidney; 5-year survival, 95%

Stage II
Tumour >7cm in greatest dimension and limited to kidney; 5-year survival, 88%

Stage III
Tumour in major veins or adrenal gland, tumour within Gerota's fascia, or 1 regional lymph node involved; 5-year survival, 59%

Stage III
Tumour beyond Gerota's fascia, or >1 regional lymph node involved; 5-year survival, 20%

Figure 15.5 (b) CT scan demonstrating a large right renal cell carcinoma with tumour thrombus involving the inferior vena cava (arrow)

Figure 15.5 (c) CT scan illustrating a left renal mass (arrow) with a cystic component. Contrast enhanced phases demonstrated tumour enhancement; Bosniak IV

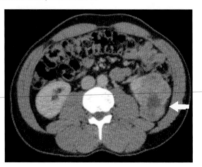

Figure 15.5 (d) TNM (Tumour (primary), lymph Nodes (regional), metastasis) staging system for renal cancer

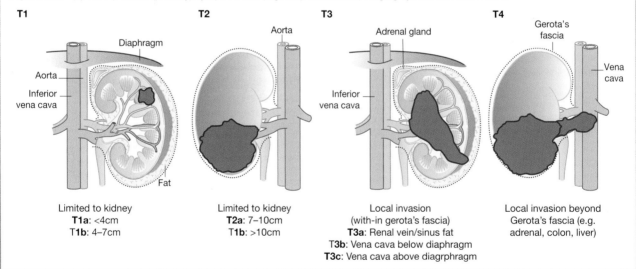

T1
Limited to kidney
T1a: <4cm
T1b: 4–7cm

T2
Limited to kidney
T2a: 7–10cm
T1b: >10cm

T3
Local invasion (with-in gerota's fascia)
T3a: Renal vein/sinus fat
T3b: Vena cava below diaphragm
T3c: Vena cava above diagrphragm

T4
Local invasion beyond Gerota's fascia (e.g. adrenal, colon, liver)

Renal cancer

One in 50 cancers are renal cell carcinoma (RCC). Each year 6000 cases are diagnosed in the UK. It affects men 1.5 times more commonly than women. It is most commonly diagnosed in the patient's sixties and seventies.

It is the most fatal urological cancer and its incidence is increasing, which may be partly attributable to the increased use of imaging modalities.

Differential diagnoses

Malignant:
- Urothelial (transitional cell) carcinoma (10%)
- Lymphoma
- Metastatic disease (rare).
  Benign:
- Simple cysts (fluid-filled sacs): 70% of all renal tumours
- Oncocytoma: 5% of all renal tumours; difficult to distinguish from RCC
- Angiomyolipoma (AML): contain fat; associated with tuberous sclerosis.

Risk factors

- Smoking
- Obesity
- Diabetes
- Renal failure/dialysis (30 times increased risk)
- Family history (including von Hippel–Lindau syndrome)
- Hypertension.

RCC is more common in industrialised countries and is common in Asian migrants to western countries, suggesting that urban dwelling or a western diet could be aetiological factors.

Presentation

- Incidentally on imaging: 50% present in this manner
- Paraneoplastic syndrome: hypertension, weight loss, pyrexia, anaemia or polycythaemia (30%)
- Visible haematuria, flank pain and an abdominal mass: <10% present with this classic **triad**
- Metastatic disease: up to 25% have metastases on presentation. Metastases may be to the lung, bone, liver, lymphatics, adrenal gland or brain
- Varicocele (rare).

Investigations

- Ultrasound: cannot diagnose renal cancer on its own but can be used as an initial screening test
- Triple-phase renal protocol contrast-enhanced CT
- Bloods: FBC, U&Es, liver function tests, calcium, erythrocyte sedimentation rate
- Biopsy: not routinely required except prior to ablation or the chemotherapeutic treatment of metastatic disease. However, cautious interpretation is required as tumours may have benign and malignant components.

Treatment

Treatment will depend on the stage of disease present and patients' co-morbidities and overall fitness.

Surgery

- *Radical nephrectomy* (open, laparoscopic or robotic): trans-/ retroperitoneal. Lymphadenectomy can be performed concurrently.
- *Partial nephrectomy* (open, laparoscopic or robotic): nephron sparing surgery can be offered to patients with small (<7 cm) tumours and/or renal failure or a single kidney.
- *Cavotomy:* removal of part of the inferior vena cava, which may require cardiac by-pass and patch repair.
- *Metastatectomy:* typically lung or, rarely, brain.

Ablative therapy

Percutaneous (using a special needle with CT guidance) or laparoscopic ablative therapies can be used for smaller tumours. They are typically employed for patients who are not fit for surgery as cancer control is less effective.
- *Cryoablation:* freezing using multiple needles.
- *Radiofrequency ablation:* high frequency alternating current burns the tumour using a multi-pronged needle.

Systemic therapy

Renal cancer does not respond well to radiotherapy or chemotherapy. Selected patients with metastatic disease may undergo a 'cytoreductive' nephrectomy. Immunotherapy is usually offered to patients with metastatic disease:
- Tyrosine kinase inhibitors (TKIs)
- Inteferon-α (IFN-α)
- Interleukin-2 (IL-2)
- Vascular endothelial growth factor (VEGF) inhibitors
- Mammalian target of rapamycin (m-TOR) inhibitors.

Surveillance

Surveillance may be offered to asymptomatic unfit patients or patients with small (<2–4 cm) indeterminate lesions, especially those with a negative biopsy.

Prognosis

The 5-year overall survival for RCC is 50%; however, prognosis is very good for patients with small tumours confined to the kidney (95% in T1a N0 M0), which are typically diagnosed incidentally (Figure 15.5). T2 disease has a 75% 5-year survival, while T3 or N1 disease is 50% and T4 or metastatic disease is <10%. Fuhrman grade and cell type (clear cell, papillary or chromophobe) are also important prognostic indicators. Follow-up schedules are individualised and typically last 5–10 years and include at least annual renal function (U&Es), chest (X-ray or CT) and abdominal (ultrasound or CT) imaging.

Figure 15.6 Bladder cancer. Courtesy of Donald Lamm

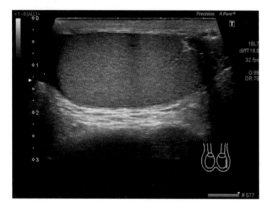

Figure 15.7 Staging of bladder cancer

Fat
Muscle
Connective tissue
Bladder lining

CIS
Ta
T1
T2
T3
T4

Figure 15.8 Invasive bladder tumour obstructing right ureteric orifice (arrow)

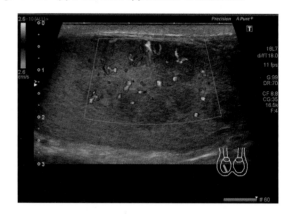

Figure 15.9 (a) Normal testicular ultrasound

Figure 15.9 (b) Ultrasound appearance of seminoma

Figure 15.9 (c) Classification of testicular cancer

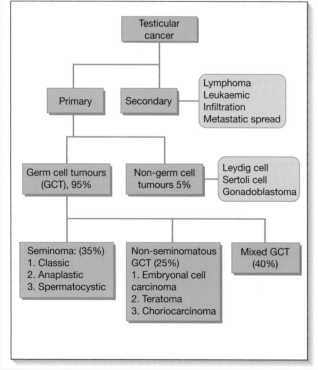

Testicular cancer

Primary — Secondary — Lymphoma / Leukaemic / Infiltration / Metastatic spread

Germ cell tumours (GCT), 95% — Non-germ cell tumours 5% — Leydig cell / Sertoli cell / Gonadoblastoma

Seminoma: (35%)
1. Classic
2. Anaplastic
3. Spermatocystic

Non-seminomatous GCT (25%)
1. Embryonal cell carcinoma
2. Teratoma
3. Choriocarcinoma

Mixed GCT (40%)

Figure 15.9 (d) Lymphatic drainage of testis

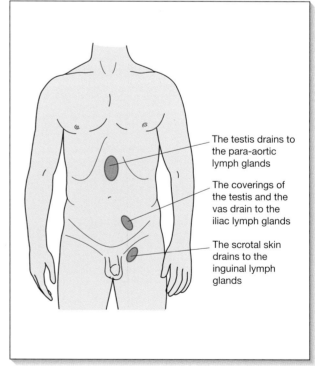

The testis drains to the para-aortic lymph glands

The coverings of the testis and the vas drain to the iliac lymph glands

The scrotal skin drains to the inguinal lymph glands

Bladder cancer

Bladder cancer is the seventh most common cancer in the UK. It has a male preponderance. There are several types of bladder cancer, but the most common type is **transitional cell carcinoma** (Figure 15.6). Other types are:

- Squamous carcinoma
- Adenocarcinoma
- Metastases.

Risk factors

- Smoking
- Occupational exposure to aniline dyes, working in the rubber industry
- Family history
- Chronic inflammation: bladder stones, bilharzia
- Radiation
- Drugs: cyclophosphamide, phenacetin, pioglitazone
- Extrophy.

Worldwide, schistosomiasis is a significant risk factor for squamous cell carcinoma of the bladder because of the chronic inflammation it causes.

Presentation

Most patients present with frank haematuria. Occasionally, some present with recurrent UTIs.

Investigations

- Flexible cystoscopy is entirely diagnostic.
- Urine cytology can be used but this does not confirm the site of the tumour as transitional call cancers can be found anywhere in the urinary tract.

Once a bladder cancer has been diagnosed the patient will then undergo a transurethral resection of bladder tumour (TURBT).

Transurethral resection of bladder tumour

A resectoscope is passed into the patient's bladder via the urethra. The bladder tumour is then cut away in chunks with a loop through which an electric current passes. The tumour is removed by washing the chunks out and samples are taken from the base of the tumour of the bladder wall to provide accurate staging.

Staging (Figure 15.7)

Staging for bladder cancer is usually in the form of cross-sectional imaging with CT or occasionally MRI. The kidneys and ureters are always imaged because of the multi-focal nature of transitional cell cancer.

Tumours are divided into two basic groups: superficial and muscle-invasive, dependent upon which layers of the bladder are involved.

Most bladder cancers are superficial (70–80%) at presentation.

Treatment

Superficial bladder cancers

- TURBT
- Intravesical chemotherapy (mitomycin c)
- Intravesical immunotherapy (BCG).

Carcinoma *in situ* (CIS) is viewed as part of superficial bladder cancer but is treated aggressively, usually with BCG as it is the precursor of muscle-invasive rather than superficial disease. BCG is thought to excite an immune response within the bladder to reduce the risk of tumour progression.

Other chemotherapeutic substances have been tried in bladder cancer such as doxyrubicin. Mitomycin C is given intravesically with a catheter either at the time of TURBT or just after, as this is when it has been shown to be most effective. It can also be given as a 6-week course intravesically for patients with multiple tumours to reduce the risk of recurrence.

Patients are usually followed up with regular cystoscopy and have a good prognosis.

Invasive bladder cancer (Figure 15.8)

- *Neo-adjuvant chemotherapy*: given before definitive treatment
- *Cystectomy*: cysto-prostatectomy in a man, anterior exoneration in a woman; removal of bladder, uterus, tubes and ovaries
- *Chemo-radiation*: external beam radiation coupled with intravesical chemotherapy.

Patients with muscle-invasive disease have a much worse prognosis, depending on the stage of their disease, of 70–20% 5-year survival.

Transitional cell carcinoma

Transitional cell or urothelium lines the whole of the urinary tract from the renal collecting system to the navicular fossa in a man.

As such these transitional cell cancers, which are predominantly found in the bladder, can occur in any site from renal pelvis to penile urethra.

This needs to be borne in mind when evaluating patients with this condition as the multi-focal nature of the condition means that they may have synchronous lesions or develop metachronous lesions at a different site within the urinary tract.

Squamous cell carcinoma

These tumours are commonly muscle-invasive at presentation, but unlike transition cell carcinomas are not normally multi-focal and do not usually appear at other points in the urinary tract. As they are poorly responsive to most chemo- and radio-therapeutic regimes, they are most commonly treated by cystectomy.

Box 15.1 Penile cancer TNM classification

T-primary tumour	
Tx	Cannot be assessed
T0	No evidence of penile cancer
Ta	Non-invasive verrocus carcinoma
T1	Invades subepithelial connective tissue
T2	Invadescorpus spongiosum
T3	Invades urethra or prostate
T4	Invades other adjacent structures

N-regional lymph nodes	
Nx	Cannot be assessed
N0	No regional nodal spread
N1	Metastasis in a single superficial lymph node
N2	Metastasis in a single superficial lymph node
N3	Metastasis in a single superficial lymph node

M-distant metastasis	
Mx	Cannot be assessed
M0	No metastasis
M1	Distant metastasis present

Figure 15.10 (a) Penile squamous carcinoma

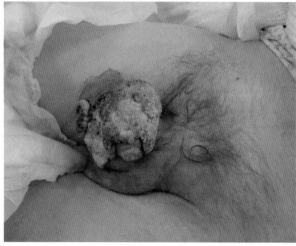

Figure 15.10 (b) CIS

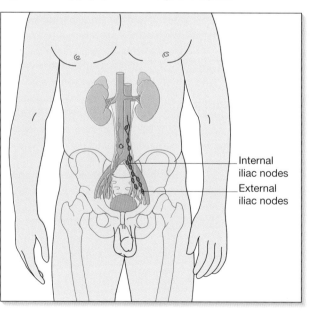

Figure 15.10 (c) Penile squamous carcinoma with CIS

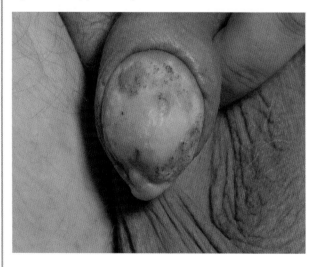

Figure 15.10 (d) Lymphatic drainage of the penis

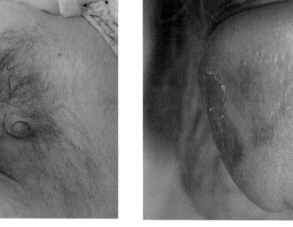

Internal iliac nodes

External iliac nodes

Penile cancer

Penile cancer is mostly squamous cell carcinoma (SCC). It accounts for <1% of all cancers among men in the UK. There is higher incidence in South America, East Africa and South-East Asia where the disease can account for 10% of all male malignancies. It occurs most commonly in men aged 60–70 years.

Risk factors

- Presence of foreskin
- Poor hygiene
- Smoking
- Exposure to ultraviolet light
- Chronic inflammation
- Human papillomavirus
- Multiple sexual partners
- Early age of first sexual intercourse.

Presentation

Most commonly, patients self present after the appearance of the lesion itself which can be associated with induration and erythema. Patients typically have phimosis which may have been longstanding. Other symptoms include pain, discharge, bleeding and storage lower urinary tract symptoms.

Examination

Examination can reveal red, ulcerated lesion or lump arising from the glans, prepuce or the shaft. The appearance can be ulcerative or papillary. Inguinal lymph nodes may be palpable.

Differential diagnosis

- Balanitis xerotica obliterans
- Leukoplakia
- Giant condyloma acuminatum
- Syphilitic chancre
- Chancroid.

Classification

- **CIS (Bowen's disease, erythroplasia of Queyrat)** CIS has all the characteristics of malignancy except for the invasion; Bowen's disease is CIS affecting the penile shaft or scrotal skin; erythroplasia of Queyrat is CIS affecting the glans or the inner layer of the prepuce.
- **SCC** accounts for the majority of penile cancers. It originates from the glans, prepuce or the shaft.
- **Other rare cancers** such as malignant melanoma, basal cell carcinoma, adenocarcinoma and sarcomas such as Kaposi's sarcoma.

Lymphatic spread (Figure 15.10)

Prepuce and shaft of the penis drains into the superficial inguinal lymph nodes while the glans or the corporal bodies drains both superficial and deep inguinal lymph nodes. The inguinal lymph nodes drain into the pelvic lymph nodes.

Distant metastasis is present in 10% of the cases at the time of clinical presentation. This can involve lung, liver, bone or brain.

Staging (Box 15.1)

Penile biopsy from the lesion is mandatory to confirm the diagnosis. Ultrasound or MRI scan of the penis to exclude corporal or urethral invasion. Staging CT of the thorax, abdomen and pelvis to exclude distant metastasis. If distant metastasis is confirmed or there is clinical suspicion bone scan may be indicated.

Treatment

Medical

- Topical chemotherapeutic agents: 5-fluorouracil or imiquimod cream
- Laser ablation
- Cryotherapy
- Radiotherapy.

Medical treatment is preserved for small CIS and low grade lesions. Patients must attend regular follow-up to assess response.

Surgical

- Circumcision for low grade lesions affecting the prepuce.
- Mohs' micrographic surgery involves excision of tissue layers carcinoma.
- Glansectomy lesions which are limited to the glans and prepuce.
- Shaft-wide local excision with primary closure or split-skin grafting.
- Partial or total penectomy. For invasive lesions involving the distal shaft and the glans penis partial penectomy with 2 cm negative margins can be curative. For lesions involving the proximal shaft, total penectomy with perineal urethrostomy may be required.

Patients who have enlarged inguinal lymph nodes at presentation are often treated with broad-spectrum antibiotics for 4–6 weeks, as in 50% of the cases the enlargement is often attributed to inflammation rather metastatic disease. Persistent lymphadenopathy, despite antibiotic treatment, should be considered as metastatic disease and bilateral lymph node dissection is recommended in those cases.

Patients with advanced inoperable disease and metastatic lymph nodes can be treated with palliative radiotherapy to delay complications (ulceration, infection) and relieve pain.

Prognosis

Penile cancer prognosis is closely related to the presence of lymph node disease. Patients with node-negative disease have a 5-year survival rate of 65–90%. Patients with inguinal lymhadenopathy have 30–50% 5-year survival rate. A lower survival rate (20%) is seen in patients with positive iliac nodes. There is no 5-year survival in the presence of distant metastasis.

Testicular cancer

Testicular cancer is relatively rare; however, it is the most common solid cancer in men aged 20–45. It is rarely seen in men below the age of 15 and above the age of 60. The crude incidence rate shows that there are 7 new testicular cancer diagnoses per 100,000 population. The survival of patients with testicular cancer has improved significantly; this is by and large attributed to the improvement and refinement of effective chemotherapy. Metastatic testicular cancer was considered as a death sentence in the 1960s until breakthrough advancement in chemotherapy and radiotherapy. Nowadays, nearly all men are cured, with a 5-year survival rate of >97%.

Clinical presentation

The most common presentation is painless testicular lump with or without gradual enlargement and heaviness sensation. However, 5% of patients with testicular cancer present with acute scrotal pain from intra-tumoural haemorrhage.

Risk factors

- Undescended testis: increases the risk by 3- to 14-fold
- Intratubular germ cell neoplasia: 50% progress to testicular cancer within 5 years
- Family history
- Exogenous oestrogen exposure during pregnancy
- Right > left: due to the increased incidence of cryptochidism on the right
- Infertility
- Caucasian men
- Higher socioeconomic status.

The risk of developing testicular cancer is highest in patients who had abdominal undescended testis and lowest in patients who had inguinal undescended testis.

Examination

A non-tender, irregular, hard, testicular lump. Scrotal skin is likely to be normal. Secondary hydrocele may be present.

Differential diagnosis

- Epididymo-orchitis
- Hydrocele
- Epididymal cyst
- Hernia
- Tuberculosis
- Syphilis.

Investigations

Scrotal ultrasound scan accurately determines whether the scrotal lump is intra- or extra-testicular. CT chest, abdomen and pelvis is also required to assess the presence of metastatic disease.

Testicular tumour markers: alpha-fetoprotein (AFP), beta human chorionic gonadotrophin (bHCG) and lactate dehydrogenase (LDH) can help in confirming the diagnosis but they can also be elevated in other conditions (i.e. hepatocellular carcinoma, lymphoma, melanoma and islet cell tumours). They can be useful in staging, prognostication of the disease and follow-up.

AFP: commonly found in NSGCT (i.e. yolk sac tumours, teratocarcinoma and teratoma).

bHCG: produced by trophoblasts. It is also commonly found in NSGCTs. However, it can also be elevated in 7% of seminomas.

LDH: can be elevated in both NSGCT and seminomas. It can help with the assessment of tumour burden in the NSGCT group.

Treatment

Radical inguinal orchidectomy: scrotal approach should be avoided as there is risk of seeding of the cancer cells into the scrotal wall.

In advanced cases with extensive metastatic disease primary chemotherapy is the treatment of choice. Depending on the response, patients may require only surveillance positron emission tomography (PET) scan follow-up or more invasive treatment such as inguinal orchiedectomy, radiotherapy, salvage chemotherapy or retroperitoneal lymph node dissection (more often performed in the USA).

Classification

Germ cell tumours

The most useful classification system for GCT is by the histologic type. It can be divided into three main categories:

1 Seminomas (35%)
2 NSGCTs (25%; i.e. embryonal carcinoma, teratoma and choriocarcinoma)
3 Mixed tumours (40%).

Seminomas are common in the fourth decade of life. bHCG may be elevated. Seminomas are radiosensitive.

Embryonal cell carcinoma: Teratoma is seen in both adults and children but more common in the third decade of life. Teratomas are radio-resistant.

Mixed cell type can include any category of the above-mentioned tumours.

Choriocarcinoma is rare (<1% of all GCT).

Metastatic spread:

- **Lymphatic spread:** (Figure 15.9d)
- **Haematogenous spread**
- **Local spread:** by direct invasion of the epididymis or spermatic cord which may result in spread to the external and/or obturator lymph nodes. Invasion of the scrotal skin or tunica can result in metastasis to the inguinal lymph nodes.

Metastasis to other organs such as brain, kidneys, adrenals, bone and lungs is seen in advanced disease. This can be as a result of lymphatic or haematogenous spread.

Non-germ cell tumours

- **Leydig cell tumour:** most common non-germ cell tumour. It has bimodal age distribution: 5–9 and 25–35 year age groups.
- **Sertoli cell tumour:** extremely rare. It has bimodal age distribution between 1 year or younger and 20–45 years. Clinically, it is characterised by testicular mass. Virilisation is often seen in children and gynaecomastia can be present in 30% of adults.
- **Gonadoblastoma:** very rare testicular tumour. Bilateral gonadectomy is recommended as the tumour is bilateral in 50% of cases. Prognosis is excellent.

Secondary tumours of the testis

- **Lymphoma:** the most common testicular cancer in patients older than 50 years.
- **Leukemic infiltration of the testis:** common site for relapse of acute lymphocystic leukemia in children. Can be bilateral in 50% of cases.
- **Metastatic tumours** are very rare. The most common primary sites are the prostate, lungs, gastrointestinal tract, melanoma and kidneys, respectively.

Further reading

Cancer Research UK. Testicular cancer risks and causes. January 2014. http://www.cancerresearchuk.org/cancer-help/type/testicular-cancer/about/testicular-cancer-risks-and-causes#factor (accessed 20 July 2016).

Cancer Research UK. Testicular cancer. November 2014. http://publications.cancerresearchuk.org/downloads/Product/CS_KF_TESTICULAR.pdf (accessed 20 July 2016).

Dieckmann KP, Pichlmeier U. The prevalence of familial testicular cancer: an analysis of two patient populations and a review of the literature. *Cancer* 1997; 80: 1954–1960.

National Cancer Intelligence Network. Penile cancer incidence, mortality and survival rates in the United Kingdom. August 2013. http://www.google.co.uk/url?sa=t&rct=j&q=&esrc=s&source=web&cd=2&ved=0CCoQFjAB&url=http%3A%2F%2Fwww.ncin.org.uk%2Fview%3Frid%3D1003&ei=ASbYU8q7JuSe7AbdioHYDA&usg=AFQjCNEMVorP-HvIaACJdxnVG7Y2Z313ng&bvm=bv.71778758,d.ZWU (accessed 20 July 2016).

Peng X, Zeng Z, Peng S, et al. The association risk of male subfertility and testicular cancer: a systematic review. *PLoS ONE* 2009; 4: e5591.

Schottenfeild D, Warshauer ME, Sherlock S, et al. The epidemiology of testicular cancer in young adults. *Am J Epidemiol* 1980; 112: 232–246.

Westergaard T, Olsen JH, Frisch M, et al. Cancer risk in fathers and brothers of testicular cancer patients in Denmark: a population-based study. *Int J Cancer* 1996; 66: 627–631.

16 Haematuria

Figure 16.1 Classification of haematuria

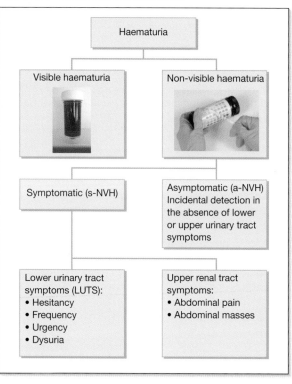

Haematuria

Visible haematuria

Non-visible haematuria

Symptomatic (s-NVH)

Asymptomatic (a-NVH) Incidental detection in the absence of lower or upper urinary tract symptoms

Lower urinary tract symptoms (LUTS):
• Hesitancy
• Frequency
• Urgency
• Dysuria

Upper renal tract symptoms:
• Abdominal pain
• Abdominal masses

Figure 16.4 CT KUB left renal stone. 48-year-old gentleman who presents with sudden onset left loinpain and haematuria. CT KUB (non-contrast) showed 14.4mm left renal pelvic stone, causing oedema of the left renal pelvis. He will indergo percutaneous nephrolithotomy

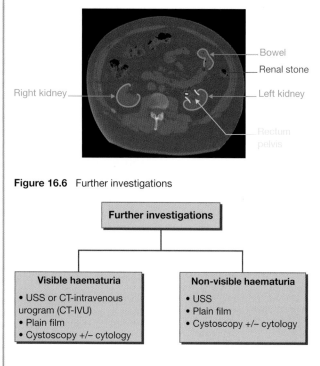

Right kidney

Bowel
Renal stone
Left kidney
Rectum pelvis

Figure 16.6 Further investigations

Further investigations

Visible haematuria
• USS or CT-intravenous urogram (CT-IVU)
• Plain film
• Cystoscopy +/– cytology

Non-visible haematuria
• USS
• Plain film
• Cystoscopy +/– cytology

Figure 16.2 CT abdomen–renal cancer. 62-year-old lady who presented with a 3 month history of cough, haemoptysis, weight loss and night sweats. O/E was found to have a right flank mass. A CT thorax abdomen, pelvis revealed a right-sided renal cell carcinoma (RCC) with pleural, pulmonary metastases and extensive inferior vena cava (IVC) thrombus. *Courtesy of Mr. D Smith, Urology Consultant at University College London Hospitals*

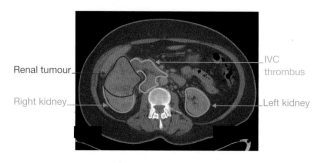

Renal tumour
Right kidney

IVC thrombus
Left kidney

Figure 16.3 CT pelvis–bladder cancer. This 73-year-old gentleman presented with frank haematuria. A cystoscopy was performed and he was found to have two large bladder tumours. He had a CT scanning and underwent TURBT to remove the tumours. Histology revealed G3 pT2 muscle invasive bladder cancer. Bladder TCC T2 NO MO

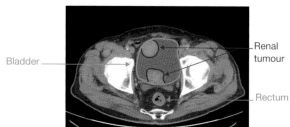

Bladder

Renal tumour

Rectum

Figure 16.5 Male urinary system and likely sources of bleeding

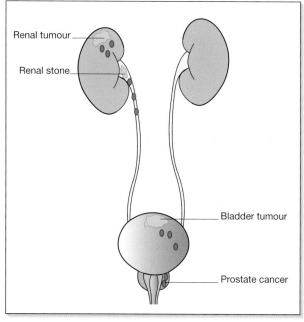

Renal tumour

Renal stone

Bladder tumour

Prostate cancer

Urology at a Glance, First Edition. Edited by Hashim Hashim and Prokar Dasgupta. © 2017 John Wiley & Sons, Ltd. Published 2017 by John Wiley & Sons, Ltd.
Companion website: www.ataglanceseries.com/urology

Haematuria is blood in the urine. The urine is coloured pink or red, or occasionally brown. There are two main classifications (Figure 16.1). *Visible haematuria,* also known as macroscopic or gross haematuria and *non-visible haematuria,* which can either be microscopic or urine dipstick positive haematuria.

Significant episode of haematuria

This is defined as:

- Any single episode of macroscopic haematuria
- Any single episode of symptomatic microscopic haematuria
- Persistent asymptomatic microscopic haematuria – 2 out of 3 dipsticks positive for microscopic haematuria.

Common causes of haematuria include urinary tract infection (2.4%), urinary tract stones (4.6%), urinary tract tumours (2.1% non-visible, 2.7% visible) and benign prostatic hyperplasia (2.5%). For other causes see Table 16.1.

Table 16.1 Causes of haematuria

Infection	Cystitis, tuberculosis, prostatitis, urethritis, schistosomiasis
Neoplasm	Renal cancer (Figure 16.2), bladder cancer (Figure 16.3), prostate or urethral cancer, Wilms' tumour
Vascular	Sickle cell disease, coagulation disorders, anticoagulation therapy
Inflammation/ autoimmune	Glomerulonephritis, Henoch–Schönlein purpura, IgA nephropathy, Goodpasture's syndrome, polyarteritis, post-irradiation
Trauma	Renal tract trauma due to accidents, catheter or foreign body, prolonged severe exercise, rapid emptying of an over-distended bladder (e.g. after catheterisation for acute retention), surgery – invasive procedures to the prostate or bladder
Endocrine	Calculi (renal, bladder, ureteric – could be due to hyperparathyroidism; Figure 16.4), simple cysts, polycystic renal disease
Drugs/toxins	Rifampicin, nitrofurantoin, senna, sulphonamides, cyclophosphamide, NSAIDs
Food	Beetroot
Others	Genital bleeding, including child abuse; menstruation; Münchausen's syndrome or fabricated or induced illness by carers

Presentation

Symptoms

- **Blood in urine:** at the beginning, middle or end of stream
- **Lower urinary tract symptoms:** storage and voiding symptoms (e.g. hesitancy, urgency, frequency – UTI, benign prostatic enlargement, bladder stones)
- **UTI:** dysuria, frequency, urgency
- **Pain:** dysuria – UTI, renal colic
- **Flank pain:** renal colic
- **Abdominal pain:** UTI
- **Bone pain:** metastatic bladder or prostate cancer
- **Abdominal mass:** renal cancer
- **Weight loss:** renal cancer, bladder cancer, prostate cancer
- **Asymptomatic.**

Signs

Hypertension: renal cancer (Figure 16.5).

Take a full urological history including palpation of the abdomen and blood pressure.

Key questions

1 Presenting complaint
  - How long have the symptoms been present?
  - Visible or non-visible
  - Haematuria at the beginning, middle or end of stream
  - Pain: loin pain, suprapubic, urethral, bone
  - LUTS
  - Abdominal masses
  - Weight loss
  - Recent trauma
  - Menstruation.
2 Past medical history
  - Any similar problems in the past?
  - Any previous investigations?
  - Parathyroid or endocrine disease
  - Coagulation disorders
  - Previous tumours.
3 Family history
  - Renal and prostate cancer
  - Coagulation disorders.
4 Drug history
  - Aspirin, warfarin, other antiplatelet or anticoagulation medications, NSAIDs.
5 Social history and occupational history
  - Smoking
  - Working with dyes or chemicals – bladder cancer
  - Recent foreign travel – schistosomiasis, tuberculosis.

Examination

- Flank and abdominal masses
- Testicular exam – varicocele can indicate renal cancer.

Initial investigations

Blood tests:

- Urea, creatinine clearance, eGFR
- FBC – anaemia.
  Urine dipstick:
- Significant haematuria is considered to be 1+ or greater. Trace haematuria should be considered negative.
- Nitrites and leucocytes – UTI.

Further investigations

- Ultrasound of the renal tract – renal masses/calculi
- A plain film of the abdomen – rule out urinary calculi
- Cystoscopy: bladder cancer, benign prostatic enlargement
- Renal angiography, CT scanning or renal biopsy are indicated in specific circumstances (Figure 16.6).

Management

Treat the underlying cause:

- UTI: antibiotics and repeat urine dipstick
- Bladder cancer: TURBT and intravesical chemotherapy
- Renal tract calculi: stone removal, ESWL
- Correction of anticoagulation disorders/therapy.

Further reading

Friedlander DF, Resnick MJ, You C, *et al.* Variation in the intensity of hematuria evaluation: a target for primary care quality improvement. *Am J Med* 2014; 127: 633–640.

NICE Clinical Guideline. Suspected cancer: recognition and referral. 2015. https://www.nice.org.uk/guidance/ng12 (accessed 21 July 2016).

Renal Association and British Association of Urological Surgeons. Joint consensus statement on the initial assessment of haematuria. July 2008. http://www.renal.org/docs/default-source/what-we-do/RA-BAUS_Haematuria_Consensus_Guidelines.pdf?sfvrsn=0 (accessed 21 July 2016).

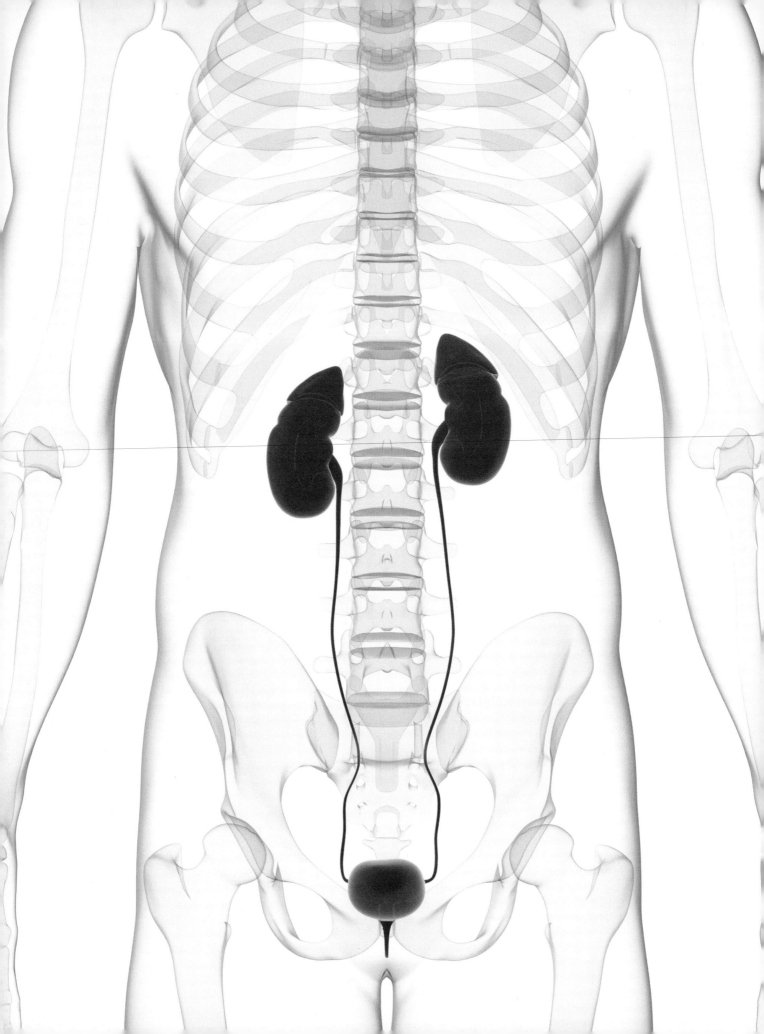

Paediatric urology

Part 6

Chapter

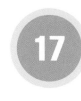

17 Common urological conditions in childhood

Figure 17.1 Picture of a foreskin affected by BXO

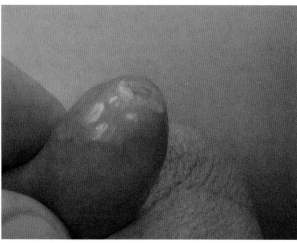

Table 17.1 Classification of hypospadias by meatal position

Location of meatus	Percentage of cases
Distal (glannular or coronal)	50%
Midshaft	20%
Proximal	30%

Figure 17.2 Classification of hypospadias based purely on meatal position

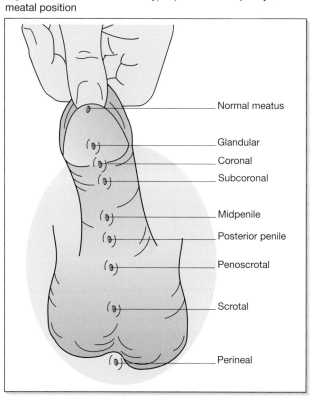

- Normal meatus
- Glandular
- Coronal
- Subcoronal
- Midpenile
- Posterior penile
- Penoscrotal
- Scrotal
- Perineal

Urology at a Glance, First Edition. Edited by Hashim Hashim and Prokar Dasgupta. © 2017 John Wiley & Sons, Ltd. Published 2017 by John Wiley & Sons, Ltd.
Companion website: www.ataglanceseries.com/urology

The foreskin

This accounts for a significant amount of non-surgical time in any paediatric urological practice. Many parents and practitioners worry that ballooning and flowering are abnormal but if the foreskin appears supple and moist then these are simply part of normal separation and development. The foreskin normally becomes fully retractile in all but around 1% of boys. Education in this area has resulted in a significant reduction in the number of circumcisions being performed for medical reasons.

The foreskin separates from the glans normally in the vast majority of boys by the age of 5 years. Anything preceeding that is most likely to be a physiological phimosis. About 10% of boys experience some delay – this may still be physiological. If the foreskin appears scarred the development of balanitis xerotica obliterans (BXO; Figure 17.1) can result in a pathological phimosis.

Mild scarring can improve with topical steroid cream but once the disease is present it can be progressive and the only way to treat it is with circumcision. Indications for circumcision are BXO and recurrent balanoposthitis. It may be useful in reducing the risk of UTIs in boys with an abnormal urinary tract. In areas where the risk of HIV is high, circumcision can help to reduce the risk of transmission.

Hypospadias

Hypospadias has an incidence of approximately 1 in 300 live male births. There are three classic elements: proximally and ventrally placed urethral meatus, hooded (incomplete) foreskin and ventral chordee. Severity has typically been classified on the basis of meatal position (Figure 17.2; Table 17.1), but it seems more likely that the ventral tissues of the penis can be much more severely affected than the meatal position suggests with a marked deficiency of the dartos, a small glans or poor glanular grove being other factors that influence the outcome of surgery.

It is important that an infant with hypospadias should not be circumcised. Discussion about surgery to reconstruct the penis includes the presence of chordee – if present surgery will be necessary to correct this. A distal meatal opening in the absence of chordee can be thought of as a cosmetic problem and therefore surgeons may be more cautious about operating. If the meatus is more proximal then this will affect the ability to stand and pass urine and later – natural insemination. The case for surgery to correct this as a functional problem seems much stronger.

Undescended testes

Testicular descent can be simplified into a two-stage process – the first occurring up to 15 weeks' gestation (under the influence of anti-Müllerian hormone from the Sertoli cells) where the testes move from the retroperitoneum (just below the kidney) to the inguinal canal. The second stage is controlled by testosterone in the latter part of gestation. The testes are normally in the scrotum at the time of delivery.

Undescended testes occur in approximately 5% of full-term male infants. This rises to 30% in preterm infants. Of these, 25% are bilateral. The strongest diagnostic criterion is a referral made at birth. In the absence of this it is important to ask the parents whether the absence of a testis was noted in the initial health checks of their son. If the answer is no then it may well be that the testis was initially present and the problem is that of a retractile testis. This is where cremasteric stimulation pulls the testis right back into the inguinal canal – careful clinical examination will demonstrate a testis that can easily be manipulated into the scrotum and will stay there. If there is doubt, asking the parents to re-examine their son while in the bath will demonstrate both testes in the scrotum.

In assessing an impalpable undescended testis it is a common misconception that ultrasound or other imaging modalities are useful. This is not the case. The most sensitive 'investigation' for an impalpable testis is laparoscopy – thus, whether present or absent on ultrasound, the child will need a laparoscopy to either bring the testis down or to be sure about its absence.

It is safe to think of the surgery in these terms – if the testis is intra-abdominal it will be brought down in two stages. If the testis is palpable (inguinal) it will usually be brought down with a single operation – inguinal orchidopexy.

Incontinence and urinary tract infections

It may seem strange to include these topics under the same heading but the principles of assessment and management bear many similarities. In incontinence it is important to understand if it is primary (i.e. the child has never been dry) or secondary (developed after a period of normal continence). In the case of primary incontinence it is essential to seek an anatomical cause but this is much less likely with secondary incontinence. In UTIs that are recurrent or complex it is important to look for an anatomical cause. The most effective way of doing this in both cases is with ultrasound.

Nocturnal enuresis (wetting the bed at night while asleep) can be monosymptomatic (i.e. not associated with any daytime symptoms). There is often no specific cause and it is common to find other affected family members. The vast majority of cases will resolve.

In patients with daytime symptoms, anatomical causes need to be considered such as a neurogenic bladder or epispadias. Functional disorders such as dysfunctional voiding, detrusor overactivity or deferred voiding can be causes.

With UTIs it is vital to have as much microbiological information as possible, both to establish the diagnosis and understand patterns of infection – is it a persistent or a recurrent infection?

In both patient sets, the taking of a thorough fluid intake and output history is very important but often incompletely carried out. This needs to be accompanied by a good bowel history. There are very often simple factors that can be changed to great effect such as the amount of fluid taken in or the frequency of voiding. Many children will vary their voiding habits on grounds such as the cleanliness of school toilets. This needs to be asked about. Many children with nocturnal enuresis will be so busy during the day they barely drink and then fluid load when they return from school – it is no wonder that they can sleep through the night without voiding or wetting. The type of fluid can also be important and in an incontinent child it can be helpful to establish a trial of drinks that are not factory-based (e.g. water, milk and natural fruit juice, especially blackcurrant juice). In both sets of patients a well-completed frequency volume chart provides a vital clue to parent–child engagement as well as firm objective information for the clinical team to work with.

Further reading

NICE. Guideline CG111: Bedwetting in under 19s. 2010. https://www.nice.org.uk/guidance/cg111 (accessed 20 July 2016).

Thomas D, Duffy P, Rickwood A (eds). *Essentials of Paediatric Urology*, 2nd edn. London: Martin Dunitz; 2008.

Wein AJ, Kavoussi LR, Partin AW, Peters CA (eds). *Campbell's Urology*, 11th edn. Vol. 4. Philadelphia, PA: Elsevier.

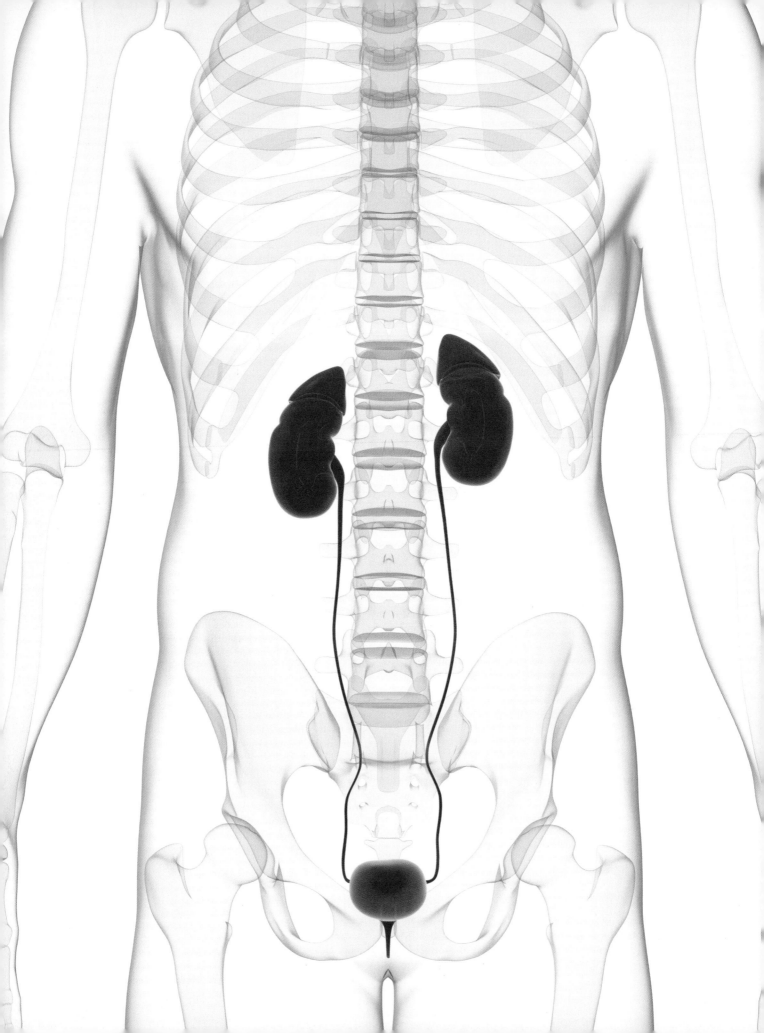

Urological trauma

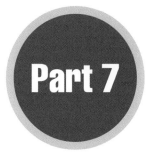

18 Urinary tract trauma including spinal cord injury

Figure 18.1 ATLS algorithm

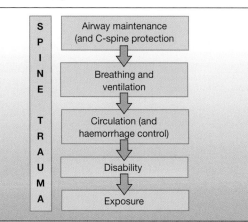

S P I N E   T R A U M A

Airway maintenance
(and C-spine protection

Breathing and
ventilation

Circulation (and
haemorrhage control)

Disability

Exposure

Figure 18.2 Assessment of the multiply injured trauma patient

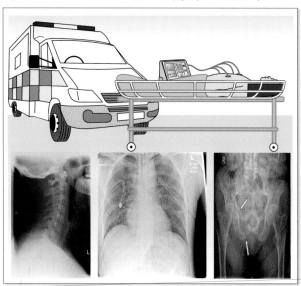

Figure 18.3 The 'pelvic' ring

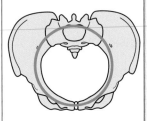

Figure 18.4 Signs of bladder/urethral injury

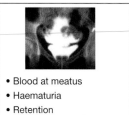

- Blood at meatus
- Haematuria
- Retention
- Perineal/scrotal bruising

Figure 18.6 Urology effects of spinal cord injury

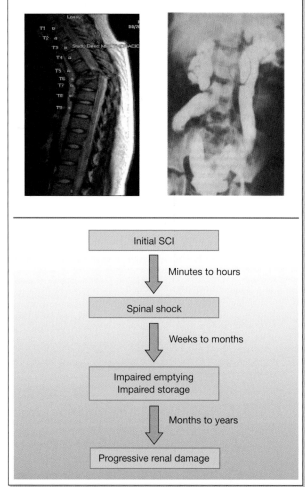

Initial SCI

Minutes to hours

Spinal shock

Weeks to months

Impaired emptying
Impaired storage

Months to years

Progressive renal damage

Figure 18.5 Tile classification of pelvic fractures

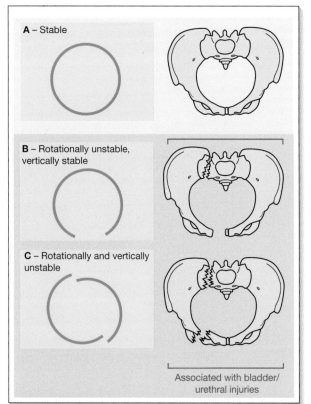

A – Stable

B – Rotationally unstable, vertically stable

C – Rotationally and vertically unstable

Associated with bladder/urethral injuries

Urology at a Glance, First Edition. Edited by Hashim Hashim and Prokar Dasgupta. © 2017 John Wiley & Sons, Ltd. Published 2017 by John Wiley & Sons, Ltd.
Companion website: www.ataglanceseries.com/urology

Major trauma

Urological trauma often occurs in conjunction with other trauma in the context of a severely injured patient. Treatment begins from the arrival of a health professional on the scene and is continued throughout the patient's journey in hospital by a multi-disciplinary team.

Advanced trauma life support (ATLS) algorithms are used in order to prioritise, identify and correct life-threatening injuries (Figure 18.1).

Cervical spine (C-spine) protection is observed throughout the initial assessment.

Trauma series

A 'trauma series' of X-rays are performed in the resuscitation room, and include an X-ray of the C-spine, chest and pelvis (Figure 18.2).

With increased access to resources, however, a trauma CT is often performed as first-line imaging. The aim is to identify early spinal, chest and pelvic injuries.

Pelvic fracture

Pelvic fractures are often caused by crush or compression injuries. Huge forces are required to disrupt the strong bony pelvic ring and associated ligaments (Figure 18.3). Associated pelvic visceral injuries (bladder, rectum, vagina) are common, as is extensive blood loss. Mortality can be as high as 20%.

The Tile classification defines the stability of pelvic ring fractures (i.e. the ability to resist physiological forces; Figure 18.5). An unstable fracture is more likely to have bladder and/or urethral injuries so signs of these should be looked for.

Urethral injuries

On examination of a patient with a possible urethral injury, the following signs should be looked for:
- Blood at urethral meatus
- Haematuria (visible or non-visible blood in the urine)
- Urinary retention (inability to void)
- Perineal, penile or scrotal bruising or haematoma.

If a urethral injury is suspected, guidelines suggest a gentle attempt can be made to insert a catheter urethrally; however, it is prudent to involve a urologist early. A suprapubic catheter may be required (inserted via on open incision) to drain the urine. The urethra can then be repaired at a later date, often at a specialist centre.

Bladder injuries

Should the bladder have been injured during trauma, diagnosis can be made by instilling X-ray contrast into the bladder and taking a series of X-ray images (Figure 18.4). Small perforations that are isolated injuries and do not connect to the peritoneal cavity (extraperitoneal ruptures) can be managed conservatively (with a catheter for 1–3 weeks). All other ruptures need to be managed surgically.

Spinal cord injury

The spinal cord is bundle of nervous tissue that runs from the medulla oblongata in the brainstem, and ends between the first and second lumbar vertebrae. It acts to transmit nervous impulses between the brain and the rest of the body and is responsible for the coordinated actions of the somatic and autonomic nervous systems. It also has a number of neural circuits that can regulate their own activity in the form of reflexes.

Spinal cord injury (SCI) prevents nervous transmission past the level of the injury. The nervous control of the urinary system is complicated with the pons and sacral cord performing different roles, which are synchronised by communication via the spinal cord.

When the spinal cord is disrupted, the bladder loses its coordinated ability to fill effectively and empty completely.

Initial injury

Immediately after SCI the nerves enter a stage of spinal shock where all reflexes are lost (flaccid paralysis). The bladder in this phase simply fills at low pressure, but is unable to contract to empty (Figure 18.6). In this phase, patients are usually managed with an indwelling catheter (urethral or suprapubic) or started on self-catheterisation.

Return of reflexes

Over the intervening weeks to months, reflexes gradually return. Providing the sacral cord is not damaged, the sacral segment begins to act autonomously to coordinate bladder filling, and stimulate emptying by causing the bladder muscle (detrusor) to contract once a certain volume is reached (neurogenic detrusor overactivity). The sphincter control mechanism is coordinated by the pons and therefore the sphincter does not relax as the detrusor contracts leading to detrusor sphincter dyssynergia (DSD). This leads to retained urine, bladder wall thickening and increases in bladder pressure which over time can cause irreversible damage to the kidneys.

Long-term urological management

The primary aim of urological management of SCI is to protect renal function. Secondary aims include maintenance of continence and bladder capacity.

Management is individualised to the patient's abilities and wishes, for example a patient with a high cervical injury and thus little hand function is unlikely to be able to perform independent intermittent catheterisation, but a carer may be able to assist with emptying an indwelling catheter.

Patients with spinal injuries require long-term urological follow-up to monitor for renal deterioration and to identify and treat common problems such as bladder stones.

Figure 18.7 Assessment of renal trauma (3% major trauma involves the kidneys)

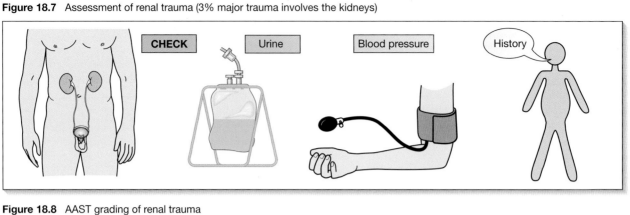

CHECK | Urine | Blood pressure | History

Figure 18.8 AAST grading of renal trauma

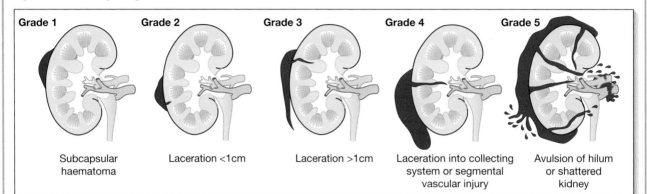

Grade 1 — Subcapsular haematoma
Grade 2 — Laceration <1cm
Grade 3 — Laceration >1cm
Grade 4 — Laceration into collecting system or segmental vascular injury
Grade 5 — Avulsion of hilum or shattered kidney

Figure 18.9 Testicular rupture

History
- Blunt/penetrating

Examination
- Haemstoma/bruising
- Swelling
- Defect in tunica

Figure 18.11 Zipper injuries

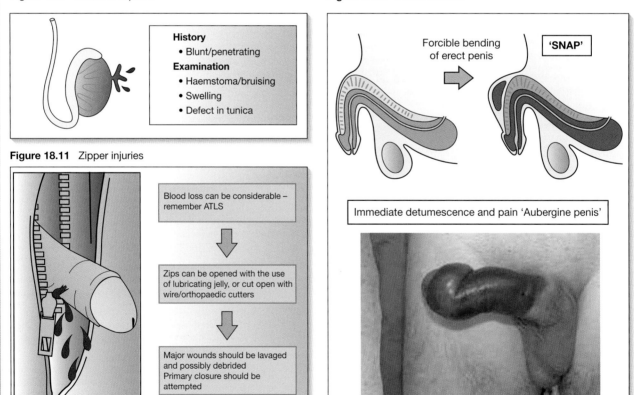

Blood loss can be considerable – remember ATLS

Zips can be opened with the use of lubricating jelly, or cut open with wire/orthopaedic cutters

Major wounds should be lavaged and possibly debrided Primary closure should be attempted

Figure 18.10 Penile fracture

Forcible bending of erect penis → 'SNAP'

Immediate detumescence and pain 'Aubergine penis'

Renal trauma

Of patients sustaining major trauma, 3% will have renal trauma. Severe injuries can be life-threatening as the kidneys receive 25% of the cardiac output and major haemorrhage can rapidly occur. Initial management should be according to ATLS principles and be performed by the trauma multi-disciplinary team.

Kidney trauma can occur from blunt or penetrating injuries and a high index of suspicion should be maintained for patients who have sustained injuries from falls or in road traffic collisions. A history of rapid acceleration or deceleration (e.g. fall from a ladder) would prompt further imaging and investigation.

On examination it is important to look at:
- The patient's urine (for visible haematuria)
- Blood pressure and vital signs readings since the injury (Figure 18.7).

Any episode of hypotension (systolic blood pressure <90 mmHg) or macroscopic haematuria increases the chance of a significant renal injury and necessitates further imaging.

The best imaging modality to evaluate renal trauma is contrast-enhanced CT which can be used to look at the vessels, parenchyma and drainage of the kidney. The indications for requesting a CT are as follows:
- Any patient with visible haematuria
- Penetrating chest or abdominal wounds
- Dipstick haematuria in a patient who has had a systolic blood pressure <90 mmHg at any point since the injury
- Rapid acceleration or deceleration injury
- Any child with visible or dipstick haematuria.

The American Association for the Surgery of Trauma (AAST) have devised a 5-point grading system for the description of renal trauma based on CT images (Figure 18.8). Renal injuries are graded 1–5 with 5 representing the most severe injuries. The majority of renal injuries are grades 1–3 (contusion or laceration, without evidence of urinary extravasation). These lower grade injuries are usually managed conservatively; patients are admitted to hospital for bed rest. Higher grade injuries (4 and 5) may need surgery if the patient shows signs of shock, or bleeding is ongoing despite transfusion. The patient may also have other injuries, and require input from a variety of specialities.

Follow-up for patients following renal trauma is essential, as there is a small risk of developing trauma-induced hypertension. The patient needs to be aware of this and needs to be monitored carefully for many years following a renal injury.

Testicular trauma

Despite their exposed location, and seeming vulnerability, testicular trauma is surprisingly uncommon.

As with all trauma, it is important to take a detailed history, focusing on the mechanism of injury (Figure 18.9). In the UK, the majority of injuries are blunt, often resulting from sporting activities (e.g. a cricket ball strike to the testis). Testicular trauma is often exquisitely painful, and accompanying nausea and vomiting is common.

On examination one should look for:
- Signs of a haematoma
- The extent and distribution of bruising and swelling
- If there is minimal scrotal haematoma a defect in the tunica albuginea may be palpable.

Unlike renal trauma, the mainstay of testicular trauma involves surgical exploration. Ultrasonography is very accurate in determining severity of testicular trauma. Although a small contusion or intra-testicular haematoma can be managed conservatively, there remains a risk of damage to the testicle from increased pressure within the fibrous tunica albuginea.

A defect in the tunica albuginea is known as a testicular fracture or testicular rupture. Surgical repair of this defect as soon as possible is advantageous for a number of reasons. It allows removal of the extruded seminiferous tubules which are likely not to be viable, but also gives the opportunity to reduce postoperative swelling by evacuating the haematoma. Early exploration and repair of the tunical defect reduces the infection rate, as well as the rate of testicular loss. There is also a theoretical advantage in that it reduces the formation of anti-sperm antibodies, and thus improves fertility.

Penile trauma

The penis is extremely well vascularised, and it is worth noting that blood loss in cases of severe trauma can be severe. Patients with serious penile trauma should be resuscitated, following the ATLS algorithm. There may also be associated injuries.

Penile fracture

Forcible bending of the erect penis can rupture the tunica albuginea of the corpora cavernosum – penile fracture. The tunica is 90% thinner in erection than in its flaccid state and hence is more susceptible to rupture.

From the history, the patient usually gives a clear story of a 'snap' or 'popping' sound, usually during sexual intercourse, accompanied by immediate detumescence and pain. The bruising is usually contained within Buck's fascia and the grossly swollen and bruised penis is sometimes said to resemble an 'aubergine'. On examination, it is sometimes possible to palpate a defect in the tunica providing that there is not too great an amount of haematoma (Figure 18.10).

With penile fractures there is a risk of a coexisting urethral injury, which would be suspected if there was blood at the urethral meatus, or on urine dipstick. Other signs include urinary retention or pain when passing urine.

Conservative management of penile fractures can lead to fibrosis and permanent penile deformity as well as increasing duration of pain. For this reason early surgical exploration and repair of tunical defects is indicated.

Zipper injuries

The prepuce can on occasion be caught within a zipper (Figure 18.11). Penile trauma is usually mild, but requires careful detangling to ensure no further damage occurs. The zipper can often be persuaded open with some lubricating jelly, but occasionally the zip needs to be cut with wire cutters in order to facilitate dismantling. In a zipper injury in a child, this may need to be carried out under general anaesthetic.

Zipper injuries should be managed as for traumatic wounds elsewhere, by lavage, debridement and attempt at primary repair, as well as consideration of tetanus prophylaxis.

Further reading

Abrams P, Agarwal M, Drake M, et al. A proposed guideline for the urological management of patients with spinal cord injury. BJU international 2008; 101: 989–994.

EAU guidelines urological trauma The EAU Urological Trauma Guidelines Panel. https://uroweb.org/guideline/urological-trauma/(accessed 20 October 2016).

Reynard J, Brewster S, Biers S. Trauma to the urinary tract and other urological emergencies. Oxford Handbook of Urology, 3rd edn. Oxford: Oxford University Press; 2013.

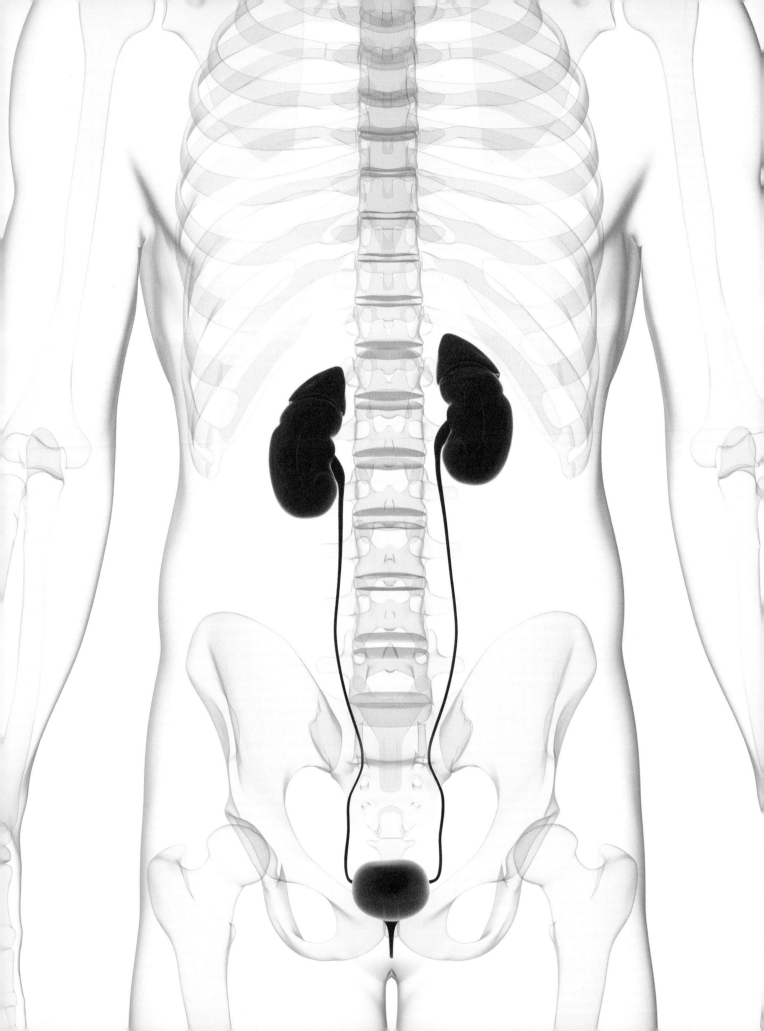

Urological procedures and equipment

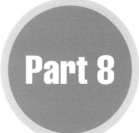

Part 8

19 Urological procedures and equipment

Figure 19.1 Anatomy of a urinary catheter

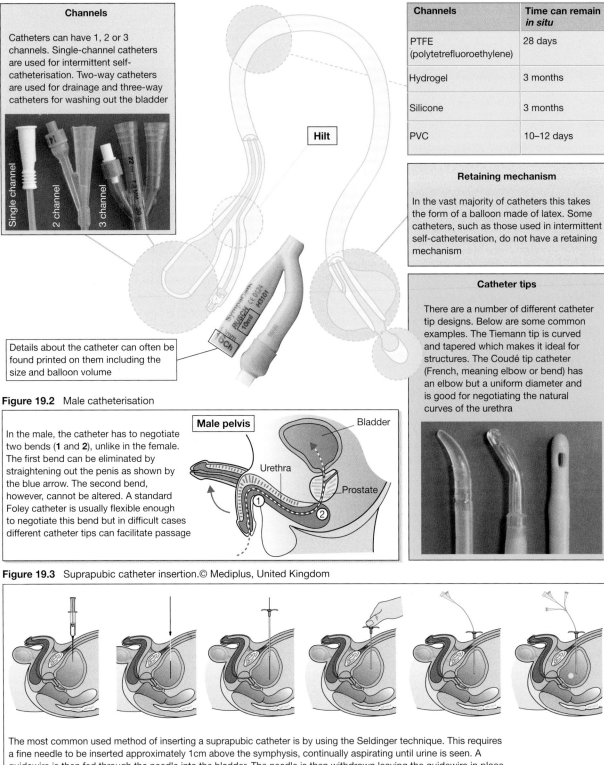

Channels

Catheters can have 1, 2 or 3 channels. Single-channel catheters are used for intermittent self-catheterisation. Two-way catheters are used for drainage and three-way catheters for washing out the bladder

Single channel
2 channel
3 channel

Hilt

Details about the catheter can often be found printed on them including the size and balloon volume

Channels	Time can remain *in situ*
PTFE (polytetrefluoroethylene)	28 days
Hydrogel	3 months
Silicone	3 months
PVC	10–12 days

Retaining mechanism

In the vast majority of catheters this takes the form of a balloon made of latex. Some catheters, such as those used in intermittent self-catheterisation, do not have a retaining mechanism

Catheter tips

There are a number of different catheter tip designs. Below are some common examples. The Tiemann tip is curved and tapered which makes it ideal for structures. The Coudé tip catheter (French, meaning elbow or bend) has an elbow but a uniform diameter and is good for negotiating the natural curves of the urethra

Figure 19.2 Male catheterisation

In the male, the catheter has to negotiate two bends (**1** and **2**), unlike in the female. The first bend can be eliminated by straightening out the penis as shown by the blue arrow. The second bend, however, cannot be altered. A standard Foley catheter is usually flexible enough to negotiate this bend but in difficult cases different catheter tips can facilitate passage

Male pelvis

Bladder
Urethra
Prostate

Figure 19.3 Suprapubic catheter insertion.© Mediplus, United Kingdom

The most common used method of inserting a suprapubic catheter is by using the Seldinger technique. This requires a fine needle to be inserted approximately 1cm above the symphysis, continually aspirating until urine is seen. A guidewire is then fed through the needle into the bladder. The needle is then withdrawn leaving the guidewire in place. A dilator with plastic sheath is run over the guidewire creating a tract protected by the sheath, large enough for a catheter (usually 16 Fr but available in most sizes as required) to be placed through and into the bladder

Urology at a Glance, First Edition. Edited by Hashim Hashim and Prokar Dasgupta. © 2017 John Wiley & Sons, Ltd. Published 2017 by John Wiley & Sons, Ltd.
Companion website: www.ataglanceseries.com/urology

Catheters

Urinary catheters have been around since 3000 BC. There have been many different designs, some of which have persisted and others that have largely disappeared from common practice.

Indications

Urinary catheters have a number of uses but the indications can be broadly divided into six categories:

1 **Drainage of urine** in urinary retention (difficulty passing urine)
2 **Monitoring** the urine output
3 **Washing out** blood from a bladder after a procedure
4 **Access** to enable substances to be instilled into the bladder
5 **Diagnostics** such as urodynamics
6 **Maintenance** of urethral lumen dimension, for example in urethral strictures.

Types of catheter

A catheter can be described in terms of its size, intended use, number of channels, tip design, material it is made from and the gender of the patient it is intended for. By considering all of these elements the correct catheter can be selected.

Size

Catheters are measured in French (Fr) or Charriere (Ch) scales (Figure 19.1). A single French unit equates to an external diameter of approximately 0.33 mm and an external circumference of approximately 1 mm. Thus, a 12-Fr catheter has an external diameter of 4 mm and an external circumference of 12 mm. Catheters commonly come in 12–22 Fr sizes. In women, a 12–14 Fr catheter is appropriate while in men, a 14–16 Fr is more suitable.

Channels

Catheters generally have one, two or three channels.
- **Single-channel:** these catheters have a single drainage channel and are usually used for intermittent drainage or urethral luminal dilatation.
- **Two-channel:** for patients who require simple drainage of urine. One channel facilitates drainage while the other allows the inflation of a retaining balloon to secure the catheter within the bladder.
- **Three-channel:** if there is significant haematuria or a requirement for continued bladder irrigation then a three-channel catheter allows saline to be instilled into the bladder via one channel while at the same time allowing blood, debris, pus and clots to flow out via the drainage channel. The remaining channel allows balloon inflation.

Tip design

There are many designs of catheter tip. The more common variants are shown in Figure 19.1.

Material

The material a catheter is composed of dictates how long it can remain in a patient without having to be changed as well as its purpose (Figure 19.1). Most catheters are made from latex (a soft and flexible natural rubber) and coated in polytetrafluoroethylene (PTFE), hydrogel or silicone. Pure polyvinyl chloride (PVC) catheters are more rigid and therefore more suitable for washing out the bladder as they resist collapse under the negative pressure generated by aspiration washouts.

Technique

Catheters should be placed using an aseptic no touch technique which avoids direct contact with the catheter by holding the plastic packaging. In men, the foreskin should be retracted and the exposed glans cleaned using an appropriate solution in a radial motion from the meatus outwards. In women, the labia should be parted to reveal the urethra and the local area cleaned in a wiping motion from the urethra towards the perineum. The patient should then be appropriately draped and a lubricating gel instilled into the urethral meatus. The urethra is about 20 cm long in the male and 4 cm in the female and ideally the amount of gel used should lubricate the whole urethra. The catheter is then introduced up to the hilt taking care to withdraw if resistance is encountered to avoid the creation of a false passage (Figure 19.2). Once urine is observed, the balloon should be inflated using the recommended volume of sterile water (usually 10 mL). The catheter should then be drawn back so that the balloon lies at the level of the bladder outlet. Care should be taken to replace the foreskin in males (if present) to prevent paraphimosis and the catheter connected to a suitable drainage bag. The procedure should be clearly documented within the notes including the volume of urine initially drained.

Suprapubic catheter

Suprapubic catheters (SPC) can be used when access via the urethra is impossible or to prevent damage to the urethra caused by a long-term urethral catheter. In many patients, an SPC will also facilitate easier catheter exchange, in particular for carers.

SPC should only be placed by clinicians with adequate training (using ultrasound guidance or endoscopic verification and the Seldinger technique; Figure 19.3) because there is a real danger of both bowel and vascular injury. Other risks include infection and pain. Patients should have a full bladder confirmed both clinically and through ultrasound observance.

Prior to the procedure:

1 The patient should be examined for lower abdominal scars that suggest adhesions and/or an abnormal bowel position.
2 The patient should be appropriately counselled regarding the potential risks, and for use of anticoagulants which are a relative contraindication.
3 Should there be any suspicion of a bladder cancer (i.e. known or haematuria), the insertion of SPC is not recommended as can lead to spread of the malignancy via cutaneous seeding.

Figure 19.4 Hopkins rod lens array. © KARL STORZ – Endoskope, Germany

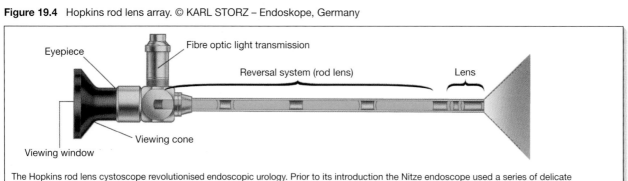
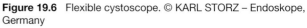

Eyepiece

Fibre optic light transmission

Reversal system (rod lens)

Lens

Viewing cone

Viewing window

The Hopkins rod lens cystoscope revolutionised endoscopic urology. Prior to its introduction the Nitze endoscope used a series of delicate lenses placed within the housing. These were prone to being dislodged and were expensive. Furthermore, the light transmission and image was poor. By using glass rods (in blue) and small air spaces that would act as 'lenses', smaller diameter, more resilient scopes were created which gave vastly improved image quality

Figure 19.5 Resectoscope © KARL STORZ – Endoskope, Germany

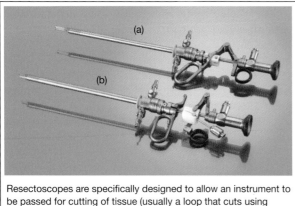

(a)

(b)

Resectoscopes are specifically designed to allow an instrument to be passed for cutting of tissue (usually a loop that cuts using electrocautery). It has two channels which allow the simultaneous infusion and extraction of irrigating fluid (a and b)

Figure 19.6 Flexible cystoscope. © KARL STORZ – Endoskope, Germany

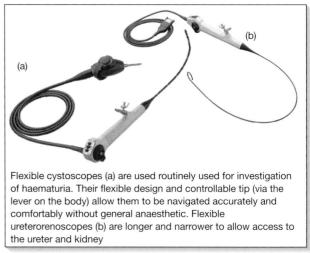

(a)

(b)

Flexible cystoscopes (a) are used routinely used for investigation of haematuria. Their flexible design and controllable tip (via the lever on the body) allow them to be navigated accurately and comfortably without general anaesthetic. Flexible ureterorenoscopes (b) are longer and narrower to allow access to the ureter and kidney

Figure 19.7 View from a distal end chip flexible ureterorenoscope of the renal pelvis and calyces © KARL STORZ – Endoskope, Germany

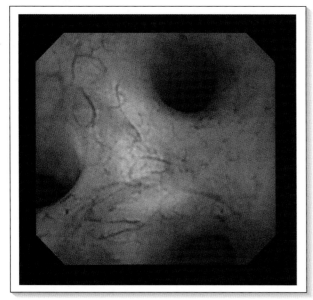

Figure 19.8 Da Vinci system. © 2014 intuitive Surgical, Inc.

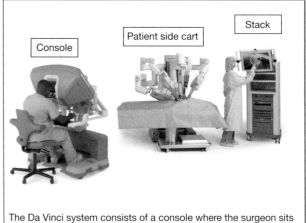

Console

Patient side cart

Stack

The Da Vinci system consists of a console where the surgeon sits and controls the patient side cart under 3D vision. The robotic arms mirror, scale and smooth the surgeon's movements and is considered a 'masterslave' system. The stack allows the assistant to see the operation as well as housing the light source and image handling equipment

Urological equipment: Part 1

Urology is an extremely varied speciality and as such is dependent on a variety of equipment. Broadly speaking, equipment can be categorised into endoscopic, laparoscopic, robotic and energy sources.

Endoscopic equipment

Urological endoscopic equipment can be classified into:

1 Rod lens endoscopes
2 Flexible endoscopes
3 Semi-rigid endoscopes
4 Distal chip endoscopes.

The choice of endoscope depends on its intended location of use. Most have either single or dual **working channels** where instruments and accessories can be inserted depending on the task (e.g. laser fibre for stone fragmentation). Other attachments include resecting loops, biopsy forceps and diathermy equipment.

Rod lens endoscopes

These are based on the Hopkins rod lens array endoscope that replaced the original scopes which suffered from low light transmittance and poor image quality (Figure 19.4). The addition of fibre optic bundles to transmit light from source to the end of the scope enabled scopes to be smaller and have a much brighter and better image. Examples of uses of rod lens endoscopes:

• **Rigid cystoscopy**: used to look inside the urethra and bladder.
• **Resectoscope**: used to perform procedures within the bladder. These allow fluid to be infused in the bladder as well as extracted (Figure 19.5).
• **Nephroscope**: used to perform procedures in the kidney via a tube placed via the skin directly into the kidney (Figure 19.6).
• **Laparoscope**: used in keyhole minimal access surgery.

Flexible endoscopes

These comprise two separate bundles of fibre optic fibres. One bundle transmits the light to the end of the scope while the other transmits the image back to the camera and operator. The bundle that transmits the image, however, must have the fibres in the same position at either end to provide a coherent image. The nature of fibre optic fibres allows light to be transmitted despite a bend in the fibre through total internal reflection which is achieved when light meets the transition between two different densities of medium (glass in this case). The construction enables internal manipulation without a reduction in brightness or image quality, not achievable with rigid endoscopes.

Examples of the uses of flexible endoscopes include:

• **Flexible cystoscopes**: used to inspect the urethra and bladder usually under local anaesthetic or with the aid of lubricating gel (Figure 19.6). The preparation for the insertion of a flexible cystoscope is the same as for a urinary catheter (see Catheters). However, the passage of the scope is performed under vision and can be directed as described previously.
• **Flexible ureterorenoscope**: used to inspect as well as perform procedures in the ureter and the kidney (Figure 19.6).

Semi-rigid endoscopes

These have the same visual mechanics as flexible endoscopes except they lack the bulky deflecting mechanism of the flexible scope and so can be much smaller. An example is the semi-rigid ureteroscopes, which are used to access, visualise and treat conditions in the ureter.

Distal chip endoscopes

A new development in endoscopy as well as laparoscopy is the use of distal chip scopes. These negate the need to transmit an image through fibre optics or lenses that degrade the image. Instead, the camera chip that receives the image is placed at the end of the scope, thereby improving the image quality exponentially (Figure 19.7).

Laparoscopic equipment

Urological laparoscopic equipment broadly consists of a screen to transmit images from the laparoscope, access port(s) to gain access into the patient's internal body cavity and an insufflator to pump non-flammable gas (carbon dioxide) to enable visualisation and instruments to perform a procedure.

Many open procedures can be performed laparoscopically with the advantages of reduced postoperative pain, smaller scars, reduced blood loss, reduced hospitalisation and quicker recovery. Although challenging for the operating surgeon, the advantages of laparoscopy have led to its widespread adoption within the field of urology.

Common urological laparoscopic procedures include prostatectomy (removing the prostate), nephrectomy (removing the kidney) and pyeloplasty (reconstructing the renal pelvis when narrowed).

Robotic surgery

The introduction of the da Vinci robotic system to many represents the next evolutionary step from laparoscopic surgery.

Developed by Intuitive Surgical, the first robot was introduced in the USA with Food and Drug Administration approval in 2000 to perform laparoscopic surgery. Since then, new versions of the system have been released with the latest being the da Vinci Xi.

The system essentially has three components: the surgeon's console, the patient side cart and the endoscopic stacks (Figure 19.8).

The surgeon's console provides the surgeon with a high definition 3D image, as well as the master controls.

The patient side cart has four arms that hold and manipulate the robotic instruments. These instruments are similar to those used in laparoscopic surgery except they are wristed which gives them seven degrees of movement and 90° articulation. The arms and instruments replicate the movements of the surgeon (master–slave) made at the console but are scaled and devoid of tremor.

The endoscopic 'stack' provides the insufflator, the light source and the images for the assistant.

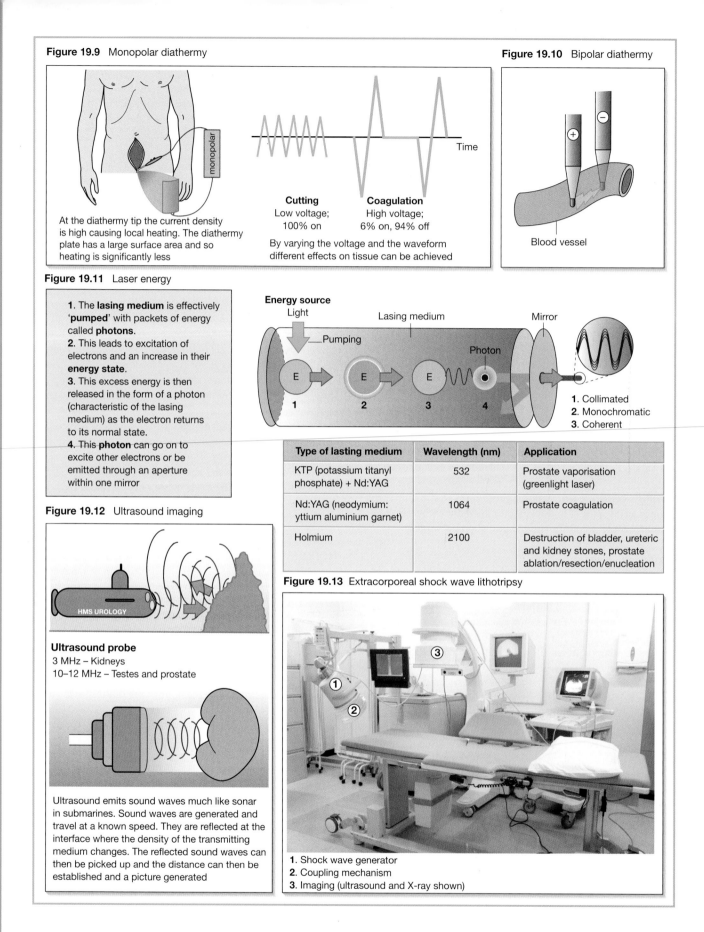

Figure 19.9 Monopolar diathermy

At the diathermy tip the current density is high causing local heating. The diathermy plate has a large surface area and so heating is significantly less

Time

Cutting
Low voltage;
100% on

Coagulation
High voltage;
6% on, 94% off

By varying the voltage and the waveform different effects on tissue can be achieved

Figure 19.10 Bipolar diathermy

Blood vessel

Figure 19.11 Laser energy

1. The **lasing medium** is effectively 'pumped' with packets of energy called **photons**.
2. This leads to excitation of electrons and an increase in their **energy state**.
3. This excess energy is then released in the form of a photon (characteristic of the lasing medium) as the electron returns to its normal state.
4. This **photon** can go on to excite other electrons or be emitted through an aperture within one mirror

Energy source
Light

Pumping

Lasing medium

Mirror

Photon

E

E

E

1   2   3   4

1. Collimated
2. Monochromatic
3. Coherent

Type of lasting medium	Wavelength (nm)	Application
KTP (potassium titanyl phosphate) + Nd:YAG	532	Prostate vaporisation (greenlight laser)
Nd:YAG (neodymium: yttium aluminium garnet)	1064	Prostate coagulation
Holmium	2100	Destruction of bladder, ureteric and kidney stones, prostate ablation/resection/enucleation

Figure 19.12 Ultrasound imaging

HMS UROLOGY

Ultrasound probe
3 MHz – Kidneys
10–12 MHz – Testes and prostate

Ultrasound emits sound waves much like sonar in submarines. Sound waves are generated and travel at a known speed. They are reflected at the interface where the density of the transmitting medium changes. The reflected sound waves can then be picked up and the distance can then be established and a picture generated

Figure 19.13 Extracorporeal shock wave lithotripsy

① ③ ②

1. Shock wave generator
2. Coupling mechanism
3. Imaging (ultrasound and X-ray shown)

Urological equipment: Part 2

Energy sources

There are a number of different energy sources used in urological surgery. The selection of the most appropriate energy source is dependent on its characteristics and the task in hand. Energy sources used in urology are electrical, light and sound.

Electrical

This is the most common energy source used in urology. It is most recognisable as diathermy or electrocautery, which can be either monopolar and bipolar. Diathermy can be used to either cut tissue or cause coagulation through dielectric heating produced by rotation of molecular dipoles in a high frequency alternating electric field.

The heat generation in electrocautery is based on Ohms' law:

$$I = V/R$$

where I is the flow of electrons or amperes, V is the force that allows electrons to flow between a positive and negative terminal and R is resistance. If the resistance is high then heat is generated.

Monopolar

In monopolar diathermy an alternating current (>200 Hz) is passed from the hand piece to the tissue where its effect is achieved and from where it then returns to the diathermy unit via an electrode plate (with a large surface area of approximately 70 cm^2) often placed on the thigh. As the current density is high at the tip of the hand piece, heat is generated. The voltage and waveform can be varied to produce either a cutting or coagulation effect (Figure 19.9).

Bipolar

In bipolar diathemy the current passes only through the target tissue between two tines of a forceps or resecting instrument. Consequently, there is no need for a 'return' plate and no damage to tissue other than that targeted (Figure 19.10).

Light

Light energy is often used in the form of a laser (**L**ight **A**mplification by the **S**timulated **E**mission of **R**adiation). Laser energy has three key characteristics:
1 **Collimated:** i.e. parallel light rays
2 **Monochromatic:** i.e. all the colours, hints and shades of a single hue
3 **Coherent:** i.e. light waves all have the same frequency.

Laser light is created by applying energy to a lasing material in a process known as 'pumping'. The energy excites the electrons within the material, which leads to the release of a packet of light known as a photon with characteristics that are peculiar to that lasing material (Figure 19.11).

The light is then transmitted to the target via a fibre optic cable. The use of a fibre optic cable allows the laser to be transmitted to its target even when the cable is flexed.

Lasers have many applications within the field of urology. They are commonly used to treat stones within the urinary tract, transitional cell carcinomas and urethral strictures, and have also been used in penile cancer and to activate certain light-sensitive medications at their target.

The most commonly encountered laser is the Ho:YAG although there are a number of different lasers employed in urology (Figure 19.11).

Sound

Sound energy has been employed in urology as a diagnostic as well as a therapeutic medium.

Diagnostic

Ultrasound imaging is based on a similar principle to that used in sonar on submarines (Figure 19.12). It relies on the creation of a sound wave through the application of electricity via small piezoelectric crystals placed in a probe. These consequently rapidly deform and create a sound wave which travels through the area to be imaged. The sound wave is then reflected back to the probe where there are changes in the density of the tissue. The reflected sound is then picked up and an image formed. There are different probes that vary in shape and frequency of sound generated depending on the organ or tissue that is being imaged. Generally, the lower frequency curved probes (3 MHz) are used for large organs and structures deeper to the skin such as the kidney or bladder, while higher frequency flat probes (10–12 MHz) are used for structures or organs closer to the surface and where more detailed imaging is required (e.g. testicles and prostate).

Therapeutic

Sound has been used in many settings within urology but most prolifically within the realm of stone disease.

Lithotripters are machines used to fragment stones by generating sound waves outside the body and then focusing them on to a point such as a stone in the kidney. They have three elements (Figure 19.13):
1 **Generator:** these create the sound wave as well as focus it. There are three main types:
  • Electrohydraulic
  • Piezoelectric
  • Electromagnetic.
2 **Coupling mechanism:** the generated sound waves need to be transmitted from the generator to the patient. This is often achieved using a gel pad although older versions used to require the patient to be immersed in a bath of water.
3 **Imaging:** this can be either ultrasound or X-ray. This allows the stone to be targeted.

Figure 19.14 Male circumcision; sleeve tachnique

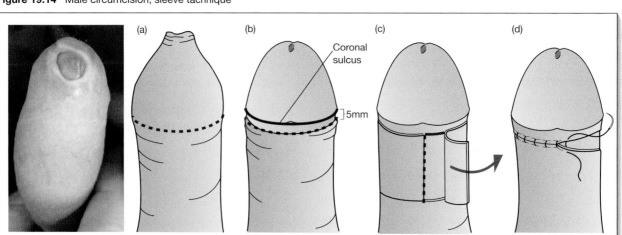

Primosis. (a) The outer side of the foreskin is incised circumferentially. (b) The inner aspect of the foreskin is incised leaving a cuff of skin approximately 5mm below the coronal sulcus. (c) A midline incision is then made between the two circumferential incisions and the foreskin is then excised. (d) The wound is then closed with interrupted dissolvable sutures

Table 19.1 Complications and risk of TURP and TURBT

	TURP	TURBT
Common	Temporary discomfort and frequency when passing urine, retrograde ejaculation, failure to improve symptoms, erectile dysfunction, infection, bleeding (sometimes requiring transfusion), need for repeat surgery, urethral stricture	Temporary discomfort and frequency when passing urine, need for additional treatment
Occasional	New finding of cancer, need to self-catheterise due to week bladder, failure to pass urine requiring a catheter, temporary/permanebt urinary incontinence	Infection. No guarantee of cure with this operation. Recurrence of the tumour or complete resection
Rare	TUR syndrome	Delayed bleeding requiring washout or further procedure, damage to the ureters requiring further intervention, urethral stricture, bladder perforation

Figure 19.15 Transurethral resection of prostate (TURP)

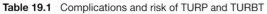

In a TURP a resectoscope is employed with a loop diathermy to take 'chips' of the prostate and ultimately create a clear channel for urine to pass through. The chips are removed through the scope with an Ellik evacuator (a type of suction device)

Figure 19.16 TUR syndrome

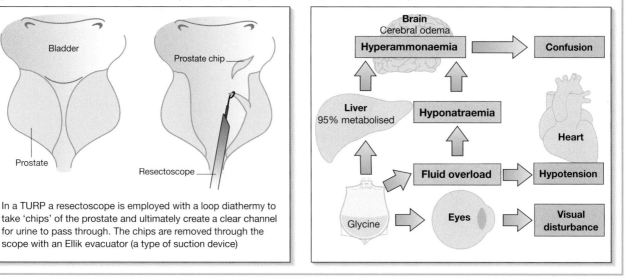

Common urological procedures

Circumcision

Approximately 30–33% of the world's males over 15 years are circumcised. It is a practice that dates back to approximately 2300 BC. In Europe, circumcision rates are declining, with male circumcision for non-medical reasons being illegal in a number of European countries.

Indications

In the UK, adult circumcision is available on the NHS for medical reasons only: lichen sclerosus, phimosis and malignancy. Consequently, the incidence of male circumcision has declined.

A drive for circumcision in areas where HIV is endemic has been fuelled by studies suggesting a 50–60% risk reduction in HIV and two-thirds reduction in human papillomavirus. Currently, the World Health Organization has circumcision clinic initiatives for low-income nations which has proved to be both effective and cost efficient.

Procedure

There are a number of surgical techniques described for adults, the most common being the sleeve technique (Figure 19.14).

Complications

Complications of the procedure include infection, bleeding (occasionally requiring surgical intervention), altered sensation, persistence of the absorbable stitches, scar tenderness, failure to be completely satisfied with the cosmetic result and occasional need to revise the circumcision when not enough skin is removed.

Transurethral resection of the prostate

Procedure

TURP involves inserting a resectoscope through the urethra and using a loop monopolar or bipolar diathermy to remove prostatic tissue in 'chips'. The objective is to remove the tissue that is impeding the flow of urine when a male is micturating (Figure 19.15).

Indications

Benign prostatic enlargement causing bladder outflow obstruction with:
1 Significant voiding lower urinary tract symptoms
2 Recurrent episodes of urinary retention despite medical therapy
3 Recurrent urinary tract infections
4 Renal insufficiency secondary to bladder outflow obstruction (high pressure chronic retention)
5 Bladder stone(s).

Complications

Complications and the inherent risks of the procedure are listed in Table 19.1.

Retrograde ejaculation is when the bladder neck, which normally prevents semen entering the bladder, is disrupted, leading to retrograde flow of semen. Patients often experience a reduction or complete absence of ejaculate on orgasm but pass it later in their urine stream. This clearly has consequences on the patient's fertility and as such patients should be carefully counselled.

Transurethral resection (TUR) syndrome is a rare, albeit potentially fatal, complication. It is caused through the absorption of 1.5% glycine that is used as an irrigant during monopolar TURP, leading to dilutional hyponatraemia. The mechanism and its clinical manifestations are described in Figure 19.16.

The time of the resection (>90 min) and size of the gland (>45 g) have been shown to increase the risk of TUR syndrome.

In the case of TUR syndrome, the procedure should be finished quickly and furosemide is commonly administered to help with the fluid overload and hyponatraemia. Intensive care admission is sometimes warranted. The correction of the hyponatraemia can be augmented using hypertonic saline although care must be taken to avoid rapid correction of sodium of >1 mmol/L as this can lead to central pontine myelinosis.

Bipolar TURP does not need glycine and isotonic normal saline can be used instead and as such is useful in patients at higher risk. Electrical energy is passed between two electrodes at the site of surgery and hence does not utilise a distant electrode.

Transurethral resection of bladder tumour

Procedure

This procedure involves inserting a resectoscope down the urethra and into the bladder. Once inside the bladder, a loop monopolar or bipolar diathermy is used to excise the bladder tumour.

Indications

TURBT is used in the diagnosis as well as treatment of bladder cancer.

Complications

The complications of a TURBT are listed in Table 19.1. One of the main complications is bladder perforation, which is classified as either extraperitoneal or intraperitoneal depending upon the location of the perforation.

Extraperitoneal perforations are relatively common and, as they do not involve the peritoneal cavity, can be managed by placing a catheter to allow drainage of the bladder for 10–14 days before removal.

Intraperitoneal perforations, although less common, are more serious. They occur predominantly at the dome of the bladder where it is at its thinnest. Fluid can be allowed to escape into the peritoneal cavity and there is always the concern that bowel has been injured. Therefore, in the vast majority of cases, laparotomy is advocated to try to identify any injuries as well as close the defect in the bladder.

Further reading

Bailey RC, Moses S, Parker CB, et al. Male circumcision for HIV prevention in young men in Kisumu, Kenya: a randomised controlled trial. *Lancet* 2007; 369: 643–656.

British Association of Urological Surgeons. www.BAUS.org.uk (accessed 21 July 2016).

Castellsague X, Bosch FX, Munoz N, et al. Male circumcision, penile human papillomavirus infection, and cervical cancer in female partners. *N Engl J Med* 2002; 346: 1105–1112.

Payne SR, Eardley I, O'Flynn K. *Imaging and Technology in Urology: Principles and Clinical Applications*. Dordrecht; New York: Springer; 2012.

Reynard J. *Urological Surgery*. Oxford; New York: Oxford University Press; 2008.

World Health Organization, UNAIDS. *Male Circumcision: Global Trends and Determinants of Prevalence, Safety and Acceptability*. Geneva: World Health Organization; 2008.

Index

Urology at a Glance, First Edition. Edited by Hashim Hashim and Prokar Dasgupta. © 2017 by John Wiley & Sons, Ltd. Published 2017 by John Wiley & Sons, Ltd.
Companion website: www.ataglanceseries.com/urology